The Management of Malignant Disease Series

General Editors: Professor M. J. Peckham
Dr R. L. Carter

1 The Management of Terminal Disease

This book is dedicated
to the memory of Gordon Hamilton Fairley

'There is a way of winning by losing, a way of victory in defeat which we
are going to discover.'

Van der Post L., (1954)
A Bar of Shadow,
The Hogarth Press, London

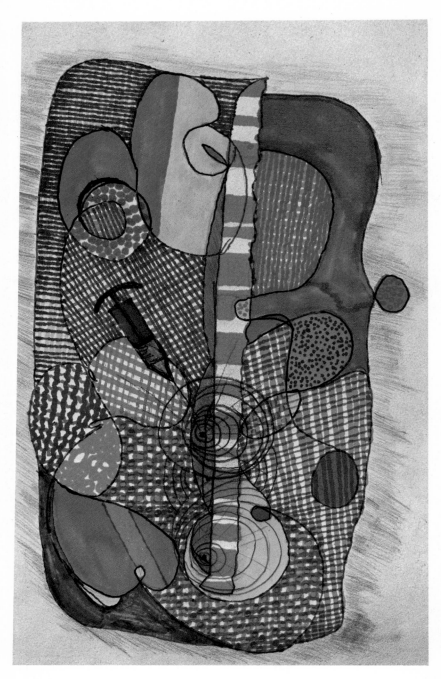

The Management of Terminal Disease

Edited by Cicely M. Saunders OBE,
MA, MD, FRCP, HonDSc(Yale)
Medical Director, St Christopher's Hospice, London

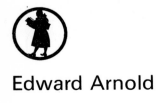

Edward Arnold

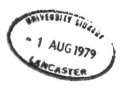

© Edward Arnold (Publishers) Ltd 1978

First published 1978
by Edward Arnold (Publishers) Ltd
25 Hill Street, London W1X 8LL

ISBN: 0 7131 4316 9

Filmset by Richard Clay (The Chaucer Press) Ltd,
Bungay, Suffolk
and printed in Great Britain by
Fletcher & Son, Ltd, Norwich

78 014804

Contributors

Mary J. Baines   MB, BCh
Consultant Physician, St Christopher's Hospice, London

Thelma D. Bates   MB, ChB, MRCS, MCRA
Consultant Radiotherapist and Oncologist, St Thomas' Hospital, London

K. C. Calman   BSc, MB, ChB, PhD, FRCS
Professor of Oncology, Department of Clinical Oncology, Gartnavel General Hospital, Glasgow

R. L. Carter   MA, DM, DSc, FRCPath
Senior Lecturer in Pathology, Institute of Cancer Research, London; Hon. Consultant Pathologist, Royal Marsden Hospital, London

M. J. F. Courtenay   MB, BCh, BAO, DObstRCOG
General Practitioner, Bridge Lane Health Centre, London

G. R. Dunstan   MA, FSA
Professor of Moral and Social Theology, King's College, University of London

Gillian Ford   MRCP, FFCM
Deputy Chief Medical Officer of Health, Department of Health and Social Security

B. Joan Haram, FRCPath
Recorder at St Christopher's Hospice

Ian McC. Kennedy   LLM, Barrister
Lecturer, Faculty of Law, King's College, University of London

Barbara J. McNulty   SRN
Lately Sister-in-Charge, Out-patients Clinic, St Christopher's Hospice, London

Peggy D. Nuttall   OBE, SRN, MCSP, DipPT
Director, Macmillan & Co. Ltd, Publishers, London; sometime Editor of the Nursing Times

C. Murray Parkes   MD, DPM, FRCPsych
Consultant Psychiatrist, The London Hospital and St Christopher's Hospice, London

D. S. Robbie   MB, ChB, DA, FFARCS
  Consultant Anaesthetist, Royal Marsden Hospital, London; lately
  Consultant Anaesthetist, St Christopher's Hospice, London

Cicely M. Saunders   OBE, MA,. MD, FRCP, HonDSc(Yale)
  Medical Director, St Christopher's Hospice, London

Robert G. Twycross   MA, DM, MRCP
  Consultant Physician, Sir Michael Sobell House, Churchill Hospital,
  Oxford; lately Clinical Research Fellow, St Christopher's Hospice, London

Thérèse Vanier   FRCP
  Medical Assistant, St Christopher's Hospice, London

T. S. West   OBE, MB, BS
  Deputy Medical Director, St Christopher's Hospice, London

Michael R. Williams   BM, BCh, FRCS
  Consultant Surgeon, Kent and Canterbury Hospital, Canterbury

Foreword

This is the first in a new series of books entitled *The Management of Malignant Disease*. It is arguably one of the most important topics to be considered – and perhaps one of the most difficult to discuss adequately between a single pair of covers. Dr Saunders brings to the subject unrivalled experience, authority and breadth of vision, and she and her collaborators have produced a book which fills a considerable need. It reflects very largely the approach adopted at St Christopher's Hospice, London and it sets out the theory and, above all, the practice which has made St Christopher's justifiably famous. Some of the material is controversial, and no effort has been made to iron out what are sometimes quite marked differences in opinion. In many instances, such differences reflect our underlying ignorance of the complex physical, mental and emotional components which make up the terminal stages of malignant disease. These areas of ignorance, and the directions in which this very new subject are likely to move in the future, are discussed; but the emphasis throughout lies firmly on practical management. As such, the book is directed to a large medical and non-medical audience who can hardly fail to gain new insights into the practice of this most exacting branch of clinical oncology.

THE GENERAL EDITORS

Preface

This book was commissioned by Professor Gordon Hamilton Fairley and the first plans completed at the time of his tragic death. Its dedication is a symbol of the hope that he, with his gifts of sympathetic and original scientific imagination, would approve its many facets.

First, an acknowledgement of my various contributors. Dr Richard Carter is a pathologist with particular interest in advanced malignant disease. This interest was expanded as a result of working for eight years as week-end clinical assistant at St Joseph's Hospice, Hackney. Professor Calman had already been involved in this area of oncology when he became the secretary of the terminal care study group to which most of the authors belong. Dr Colin Murray Parkes has been concerned with the needs of the bereaved for more than twenty years and was involved with the planning of St Christopher's Hospice from 1965. Since its opening in 1967 he has spent one or two days weekly among its staff and patients and has directed its psychosocial studies. After ten years' experience in general practice, Dr Mary Baines joined the clinical team of St Christopher's Hospice shortly after the opening. She has developed the daily work of the wards and has also studied the underlying causes of the physical distress which brings over 600 patients a year to the Hospice. She joined Mrs McNulty in pioneering its domiciliary service, the first such team to be based in a hospice unit. Dr Robert Twycross first made contact with me at St Joseph's Hospice while he was still a medical student and it was a common, continuing interest which drew him to St Christopher's Hospice in 1971. He was invited to undertake comparative studies of diamorphine and morphine as Clinical Research Fellow, supported by the Department of Health and Social Security and the Sir Halley Stewart Trust. This was a development of work on the use of narcotics in terminal care, first observed at St Luke's Hospital, London, and later developed at St Joseph's Hospice in the 1950s and 1960s. Dr Robbie, who had opened the Pain Clinic at the Royal Marsden Hospital, was invited to St Christopher's Hospice to perform nerve blocking procedures as needed, but he was also invaluable to us as a sounding board for ideas and a perceptive external critic. In years past, Mr Michael Williams and I met on Mr N. R. Barrett's firm at St Thomas' Hospital, as houseman and medical social worker. In due course Michael Williams became a Consultant Surgeon at Canterbury and, in his capacity as Surgical Tutor, organized two symposia on Pain and the Care of the Dying, in which I and other members of the staff of St Christopher's Hospice took part. It was Mr

Barrett who first directed me from nursing and medical social work to medicine: 'It's the doctors who desert the dying . . . go and read medicine . . .'. He aroused a similar interest in his houseman. Dr Thelma Bates always visited any of her patients who had been transferred to the Hospice. When the need for a closer look at the common ground between cytotoxic chemotherapy and terminal care first brought Dr Therese Vanier to join our team part-time, it soon became obvious that there should be a consultant in radiotherapy combined with chemotherapy. Dr Bates has been a regular consultant at the Hospice since 1974.

This group of authors present the different clinical fields which form the background to the chapters describing a more general approach to terminal care. Dr Thomas West has extended our involvement with the families of our patients ever since he returned to this country after 12 years in the more closely knit society of Northern Nigeria, and has stimulated the development of our ward meetings and teamwork. Mrs McNulty pioneered the work of St Christopher's Hospice among families in the neighbourhood by consulting with and working alongside the doctors and nurses in the local family practices. Miss Nuttall, formerly editor of the *Nursing Times* and a Night Sister in a London Teaching Hospital, and Dr Michael Courtenay, General Practitioner and Course Organizer of the St Thomas' Hospital Vocational Training Scheme for General Practice (Vice-President of the Society for Psychosomatic Research), were asked to comment on the work described from their position outside the special centres and on its relevance to general hospital and family practice. They have not hesitated to underline some alarming differences in standards.

Professor Gordon Dunstan is one of three Hospice Council members who have contributed. His insistence on studying ethics, not in philosophical abstraction but among practitioners, brought him as a learner into the medical field.

Dr Joan Haram has worked as a volunteer member of the team since the beginning. Her meticulous and untiring work as recorder has established a unique set of records and retrievable information.

Dr Gillian Ford's chapter is her personal view. For many years before terminal care became one of her concerns at the Department of Health and Social Security, she had also been one of St Christopher's volunteer doctors, spending a week-end a month as the only doctor on duty.

Mr Ian Kennedy has written elsewhere on this subject and we have had the pleasure of correspondence and visits with him over the past few years.

Mention is made in the text of other works in this field: those on whose experience St Christopher's has drawn and others who have entered the field since the Hospice opened. One patient has contributed directly and innumerable patients and their families and ward staff, indirectly.

I am deeply indebted to all the contributors for their hard-work and patience; to Mrs Mary Smith for endless retyping of early drafts, Miss Jenny Jameson for dealing with mountains of correspondence and Mrs Christine Kearney for the final drafting; and to Edward Arnold (Publishers) Ltd and the tolerance of Mr Paul Price and Miss Barbara Koster.

London, 1978   CS

Contents

1

Appropriate Treatment, Appropriate Death

Cicely M. Saunders

'And a certain woman . . . had suffered many things of many physicians, and had spent all that she had, and was nothing bettered, but rather grew worse'
  St Mark's Gospel 5:25, 26

'There is a general understanding that terminal care refers to the management of patients in whom the advent of death is felt to be certain and not too far off and for whom medical effort has turned away from therapy and become concentrated on the relief of symptoms and the support of both patient and family.'
  (Holford, 1973)

That nothing can be done to arrest the spread of tumour does not mean that there is nothing to be done at all. One important support to everyone concerned will be adequate treatment of the physical distress of dying. The control of individual symptoms is becoming increasingly sophisticated and the question 'What is the relative value of the various available methods of treatment in this particular patient?' (Cade, 1963) is as pertinent now as at any stage of a patient's illness. It is imperative that we recognize the moment when 'therapy' or 'active treatment' is becoming irrelevant to the needs of a particular patient. Some recent advances make such decisions increasingly difficult. Terminal care is a facet of oncology, concerned with the control of symptoms instead of with the control of the tumour. There is an increasing overlap between these two parts of the total discipline, and it is important that all the doctors concerned should be aware of the possibilities of each and judge together what is appropriate for every patient. There are, as it were, two 'systems' which are shown diagrammatically in Fig. 1.1.

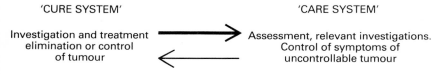

'CURE SYSTEM'   'CARE SYSTEM'

Investigation and treatment   ⟶   Assessment, relevant investigations.
elimination or control   Control of symptoms of
of tumour   ⟵   uncontrollable tumour

Fig. 1.1. 'Cure' and 'care' systems.

As active treatment becomes irrelevant the movement may be mainly towards 'Care', but no patient should become locked irretrievably in what is (or may become) for him the wrong system. The aims of the two are not mutually exclusive, and effective control of symptoms may accompany or revive the prospect of further treatment. The overlap referred to is shown in Fig. 1.2.

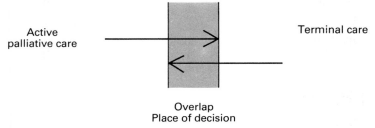

Fig. 1.2. Overlap of the 'cure' and 'care' systems.

We tend to consider only the doctors' decisions, and patients and families are frequently informed afterwards rather than being involved in them. Some patients certainly appear to take no interest in the changes being made in their treatment; others demand that 'everything possible should be tried', without question as to likely side-effects or chances of benefit. Some offer, with a certain bravado, to have any new treatment 'tried out' on them. Others immediately despair when they suspect cancer and do not present until obliged to do so by advanced, totally incurable, disease.

Yet there are surely many who could and should be involved more often. Does the 'place of decision' involve the doctor only? A woman may, for example, decide to forego further surgery or a course of radiotherapy which would keep her away from home while her children are taking important examinations. Should she not be included in the team making the decisions? People who come to us for treatment sometimes do not realize how much control they have given us; do they always intend to abrogate so much responsibility?

Another definition?

Unhappily, the terminal stage could also be defined as beginning at the moment when the clinician says, 'There is nothing more to be done,' and then begins to withdraw from his patient. Patients are well aware when this happens and, on their admission to a unit such as St Christopher's Hospice, they reveal this with sad clarity.

'To imply that nothing helpful can be done is inexcusable and seldom if ever true' (Smithers, 1960). Nor do we always realize how much we can do simply by coming to see the patient even though we have nothing to offer in the (by now) irrelevant context of radical treatment. We fail to understand what patients with terminal disease ask of us. They are commonly too realistic to expect that we can take away the whole hard thing that is happening to them; instead they ask for concern and care for their distress and symptoms. Above all, they ask for our awareness of them as people. At no time in the total care of the cancer patient is this of greater importance (see Chapters 4 and 10).

Hinter (1963) described the high incidence of physical and mental distress among patients dying in the wards of a teaching hospital, revealing how much we need to learn and to teach before the proper standards of relief reach every patient. We should aim for the relief that enables a patient not only to die peacefully, but also to *live* until he dies, as himself and not as what has been termed an 'uncomplaining residue' (Weisman and Hackett, 1962). He can hardly be involved in any decisions while he is either swamped by distress or smothered with treatment. We need to be concerned with the quality of living, hard though it is to judge this for another person. At the same time, while we are aware of the possibility of regression even at this stage (and may well share this slender hope with our patient), we have to see that this part of our care (even though it ends with the patient's death) is both positive and important in its own right.

Successful symptomatic treatment should enable a patient to be so relieved of physical distress that he is freed to concentrate on other matters. If we are to overcome the sense of failure which tends to pervade the atmosphere which surrounds the dying, we need to be aware of the proper criterion of success in this situation. It is not to be seen primarily in our activities but rather in what the patient and his family can achieve in the face of progressive physical deterioration. This may be the most important part of his life, and the spirit often becomes stronger and more individual as the body weakens.

Management of terminal disease presupposes an informed decision that active therapy is now inappropriate—and the patient and his family may have some part both in giving information and in the decision itself. Such management will include everything which will help the patient to find his own way of dying, his own death. Weisman has called this process 'safe conduct' and has developed the concept of an 'appropriate death' (Weisman and Hackett, 1962; Weisman, 1977). He defines it as 'an absence of suffering, preservation of important relationships, an interval for anticipatory grief, relief of remaining conflicts, belief in timeliness, exercise of feasible options and activities, and consistency with physical limitations, all within the scope of one's ego ideal' (Weisman, 1977). The preservation of important relationships probably requires a certain sharing of truth and may mean that both the patient and the one he is leaving will grieve—alone and together—in anticipation of their parting. I have seen many times that such anticipation can facilitate the resolution of conflicts (though, as Parkes points out, it may also exacerbate them; see Chapter 4). Our own experience is more often of a positive outcome. Such final resolutions, together with a feeling of completeness and fulfilment, can make this the 'timely' moment to die, even for someone whose age or responsibilities would seem to make this improbable. We may have different ideas concerning the meaning of our life and death, but we can all try to help a patient to attain some kind of harmony with what he sees as truth and rightness. Our own continual experience and the challenges to our beliefs and their rethinking in our daily experience may help to encourage such progress in our patients. Words are rarely needed, and may hinder this essentially individual process.

Such preparation for death is possible for those without a sense of any existence beyond this world as well as for individuals who believe in some form of immortality and a God into whose hands they may commend their spirits. All humanity shares apprehension of any unknown—most of all the unknown of death. Religion in itself does not make death easier, certainly not if it is merely seen as a somewhat magical way of avoiding trouble. Religion is not a way of manipulating the world, but rather a way of responding to the world. It is widely held that true faith is rarely met today; but our experience is that many people and their families show quiet confidence and simple faith in unseen Love. We also recognize the creative endurance of those who believe that their suffering has been given meaning by something or someone beyond them- selves. These beliefs do not avoid the pain of parting but can greatly assuage its anguish.

Whatever our own beliefs, we should never impose them on another person, least of all on any individual who is dependent upon us. But anyone who is trying to live in response to the demands his own life makes upon him, whether he sees this in any kind of religious terms or not, can create a climate in which another may find the strength to reach out trustfully and say 'Yes' to life and to death.

Appropriate truth?

Truth is not merely a matter of words and we are likely to find the particular truth which is fitted to our patient's need only in some kind of relationship with him. This question is discussed in Chapters 4 and 10, but it bears so directly upon the decisions discussed above, on the whole management of a terminal illness and on all the relationships involved, that it seems appropriate to consider some of the arguments in the continuing debate which surrounds the question of 'telling'.

It is common form to tell a patient little or nothing about his condition but to put the family fully into the picture. What do we do to our patient and to his relationships with his family and friends when we create this kind of barrier of unshared truth between them? A man describing his illness to me said: 'I couldn't think what had happened to my marriage. What had I done that I should suddenly feel so separated from my wife, why was she obviously so sad and anxious?' When his disease recurred, he extracted the truth from the doctors at his treating hospital. I subsequently asked him, 'Back at the begin- ning, would you rather that your wife had been told less or that you should have been told more?' The patient answered, 'The first—but at least we should have been together.' He had responsibilities, too.

We hesitate to tell the full truth to a patient who is living appropriately, believing his illness, though perhaps serious, is not fatal. Here it may well be kinder to withhold its full implications from the family as well. We can suggest that it would be wise not to undertake new and heavy commitments at this stage without implying that the patient is already mortally ill. There are times when we can honestly say that we do not know precisely how the disease is progressing and take a more optimistic viewpoint. However, when the patient's confidence in recovery is being undermined by the processes of illness and the impairment of communication with those nearest to him, then the unknown is often more fearful than the most dreaded reality; and it is likely that the time has come for a more frank discussion. This should not be forced nor will it necessarily give the full truth of the situation, as the doctor sees it, delivered at one blow; rather, it shows the clinician's readiness to follow the patient's questions and observe any verbal or non-verbal clues he may give. This is one of the aspects of terminal care which each doctor discovers in his own experience if he is prepared to listen, without any prepared answer or technique, and to respond to each person as he feels it right at the time. Those who see a patient once in consultation may be able to do this helpfully, but we should never assault another person with a truth which he is not yet ready to handle. The doctor who allows or encourages open interchange should normally be the one who can promise that he will never abandon the patient and who gives the assurance that he will control any physical distress and will discuss and exploit any improvement. He also needs to say that he will share this knowledge with the family and suggest that they can now discuss it together. Some families resist this strongly and try hard to 'protect' the patient. They may sometimes be right, but they are not always the best judges, being much oppressed by their own anxiety, and every effort must be made to support them as well. It is hardly surprising that if a family is asked whether a patient should be informed at the first moment of their shock at being told of a fatal prognosis, that their immediate reaction should be that the truth should be kept from him. Nor, later on, that the pain the knowledge is causing them should make them wish to protect the patient from enduring it also. But we meet many patients who have suffered alone with the very truth from which all around them were persuading themselves they were protected. It is possible, as Dr West describes in Chapter 10, to help such a family move from an entrenched position of denial and share at least some of the last part of their life together. Joint discussions are often helpful and the patient may at times be the strongest member of the group (Chapter 4).

Doctors may mistrust such openness but if they speak with care, beginning with somewhat open-ended or even ambiguous remarks, they will learn to judge how much to say at any one time. This demands all we can give of our time and our sensitivity, but opportunities will come for those who have confidence in their patients' courage and common sense—qualities which do not disappear along with good health (see Chapter 4).

It is seldom appropriate to present full information without testing out the patient's expectations in some way, but I remember giving an unequivocal answer to a man. It would have been an insult to his courage and determination to have done anything else. He asked, 'Was it hard for you to tell me that?' When I replied 'Yes—it was', he said 'Thank you. It is hard to be told but it is hard to tell too,' and repeated 'Thank you'. We have to watch what people do with the truths we give them, and I had no cause to regret this unusual directness. I believe his answer also tells us that if it is *not* hard to tell, then we should hesitate before doing so, for it is a serious commitment from one person to another. Some patients deliberately avoid asking questions or receiving information and others are reported as reacting adversely to such news. Such silence must be respected but at times one is tempted to ask, 'But *how* did you tell him?' or 'What did you let him tell you?' (see Chapter 4). These questions are not always justified—we have all made great efforts to help and still judged incorrectly. It is a comfort to know that many people who do not wish to be led into facing reality are capable of 'forgetting' an entire conversation of this kind. The human mind has an invaluable capacity to repress an unpleasant truth.

Several investigators have shown that many more people are aware of their diagnosis and prognosis than those around them realize. Hinton (1963) carried out a controlled study of a group of dying patients in the wards of a London teaching hospital. He showed that 50 per cent of his 102 dying patients already had a shrewd idea of the severity of their illness when he first interviewed them and that 'Awareness of dying grew so that three out of every four spoke of this possibility or certainty'. These patients had not been 'told' and the ward staff were often unaware that they had this knowledge. Weisman and Hackett (1962) have studied the knowledge of their diagnosis and prognosis held by groups of patients. Almost all those with heart disease had been given full information on both points while only 7 of 20 cancer patients were so fully informed—though a further 10 had been given some information. On questioning these two groups, Hackett and Weisman found that only 9 of the 20 patients with heart disease were fully aware, while 10 of the 20 patients with cancer were said to have 'full knowledge'. A similar study of children with leukaemia for whom a massive effort had been made to conceal the facts showed that 96 per cent were aware of what was happening and its implications. People acquire knowledge by various means, and deception fails more often than we suppose. Weisman (1972) discusses this carefully in his book *On Dying and Denying*. Patients are quick to sense to whom it is safe to talk. The more secure a patient feels the more likely he is to ask questions or to feel his way tentatively towards talking freely.

The real presence of another person is a place of security. I recall remarking to two psychiatrists that when patients are in a climate of safety they will come to realize what is happening in their own way and not be afraid. One said: 'How can you speak of a climate of safety when death is the most unsafe thing that can happen?' To which the other replied: 'I think you are using the wrong word. I think it should be "security". A child separated from his mother may be quite safe—but he feels very insecure. A child in his mother's arms during an air raid may be very unsafe indeed—but he feels quite secure.' We have to give all patients that feeling of security in which they can begin, when they are ready, to face unsafety. This may not necessarily be the knowledge of their approaching death. It may be apprehensions concerning investigations or treatment, changes in the situation, hospital admission, or the acceptance of increasing weakness. *Security does what deception or denial cannot do.* It may protect a patient from knowledge of the real issues entirely, and it can certainly help to lighten much of the burden of that knowledge for, above all, it relieves that isolation which accentuates all suffering.

Although bad news given starkly can have devastating results, knowledge of a fatal prognosis does not in itself inevitably lead to apathy or despair. There is clinical evidence of such knowledge 'galvanizing a will to live' which was not apparent before. 'Untapped potentials for responsible and effective behaviour as well as less depression and blame for others became evident. Honest and sensitive talk . . . tends to attenuate feelings of guilt and inadequacy not only in the patient but also in professional personnel and family as well' (Feifel, 1977). Truth and hope are not mutually exclusive, and the informed patient is frequently better able to fight for his life because he knows the real battlefield. Surely most of us wish to take some responsibility for our dying as well as for our living?

Inept words cannot be unsaid but they can be softened or forgotten, such is man's capacity for denial. We shall learn to do better if we examine our own mistakes and continue to visit the patient and help him as best we can within his own frame of reference. Only occasionally does one have to withdraw completely. We should remember that our sins of commission—too much told and too soon, or a rash answer given to another doctor's patient without previous discussion—will be visited on our heads many times; our sins of omission—our neglect of the isolated, frightened patient who can gain no real reassurance—are not usually apparent and we rarely receive the blame we then deserve.

Many of us have seen the kind of hope that springs out of realization, from facing and tackling a situation, however bleak that situation may be. Much trauma would be avoided if, as Parkes points out in Chapter 4, we realized that a large element of the defensiveness which surrounds a patient is unnecessary and self-defeating. Most dying patients are aware that time is running out, whether or not the staff looking after them are willing to acknowledge it or the family can face talking about it (Weisman, 1972).

Yet, having said all this, we must remember that love does not always need words to convey its meanings and that a family may share these problems and say their farewells in silence. Doctors or nurses, too, can give their support without direct discussion. Talk of symptoms, which may be used as a way out of involvement with such problems, can also be a way of meeting a patient with reassurance on a much deeper level.

West points out in Chapter 10 that the time of admission may provide a crucial opportunity to bring reality into a family separated by deception. Contrary to much belief, although some patients choose to come because they know what to expect from past family experiences, many people do not associate St Christopher's Hospice solely with death. Its mixed group of patients, the wing for elderly residents, its discharges and the Home Care and Outpatient service enable those who come to us for admission to identify with any of these groups. Some who did not realize how ill they were will move gradually towards truth, often asking questions or making oblique comments to students or members of staff (whom they know are not in a position to give answers) until they are ready to approach the doctor. Recording a patient's comments on the pink sheet in our notes (see p. 145) helps the ward team to share their knowledge of the patient's feelings; it also sharpens their perceptions. If we believe that it is possible to allow open communication it does not mean that this will necessarily take place. Words are often unnecessary, and one-half of St Christopher's pink sheets are empty—not only because a busy staff has failed to record something. It does mean that all conversations are more relaxed and arise spontaneously out of a personal interchange. Although there are teams whose declared policy is not to tell the truth (McIntosh, 1977), most patients finally realize what is happening even if they prefer not to talk about it (Hinton, 1974; Witzel, 1975). Mrs S., aged 40, in hospital for a radical mastectomy, found herself in the bed next to someone of her own age who was dying with metastatic breast cancer. This patient had increasing pain and paralysis and spent much of her time watching the clock, waiting for her next injection. As Mrs S. described it, 'Everybody knew she was dying—and took a step back. She was encouraged to pin all her hopes on a visit from the

Consultant and in some new treatment that he might suggest—at length he arrived, but his visit came too late, she was already unconscious.' Mrs S. wrote to me, 'Her last three weeks were spent anticipating that visit—to my mind they would have been better spent on more important things than false hopes. I'm convinced that she would have preferred the truth and that the people who were nursing her had passed the buck.' Mrs S. said to a group of students, 'I think "hope" is almost a dirty word to me now.' In discussion she added, 'I can face dying, I can face pain, but what I can't face is being treated as less than a person.'

The various fears associated with advanced cancer in the public mind include fear of pain, of pain-relieving drugs which will both swamp personality and inevitably lose their effect, of dependence and isolation and of 'being kept alive by technology' without having any choice in the matter. In this book we are concerned to erase these fears and to present general principles of analysis, assessment and treatment which can be interpreted in any setting and for each individual patient. This has been a largely unexplored field—'an aspect of oncology whose scientific foundations are only just beginning to be laid' (Symington and Carter, 1976). There is still much to be learned of the natural history of advanced disease and the pathological processes at work (see Chapter 2), the basis for specific symptoms is often imperfectly understood, and treatment is haphazard or at best empirical (see Chapters 3 and 6). Myths concerning the use of analgesics, especially the narcotics, still deny relief to many patients (see Chapter 5). Neither patient nor family receives the emotional and social help which concerned professionals of many disciplines (and volunteers) could offer them (see Chapters 4 and 10). The contributions which radiotherapy, chemotherapy and surgery can make in the care of unremitting disease are only infrequently considered (Chapters 7, 8 and 9). Often, patients say that they wish to die in their own homes, and many families feel disappointed and guilty when lack of adequate support makes this impossible (see Chapter 11).

We have tried to draw together on our practical experience and records to present a guide to clinical practice in this field and to look at the mental and social needs of patients with terminal disease. As well as aiming at the highest medical standards, we must consider the philosophy, ethics and theology of our practice (see Chapters 13, 14 and 15). If we are to have the strength to 'watch' with a patient and family in distress and anguish, we have to look to our own beliefs and our own supports (see Chapter 15). The phrase 'watch with me' comes from the story of Jesus facing death in the Garden of Gethsemane (St Matthew's Gospel, 26:38) sums up the deepest need of any person facing death or desolation. It did not mean 'Take away', it could not have meant 'understand or explain'—its simple and costly demand was to 'stay there'. We can offer this as we work for the 'good death' which is a major factor in the continuing life of the surviving family; it is also the incentive and reward of good terminal care.

> 'I've heard illness out
> Until it has nothing to say to me,
> And I thank God I have the last word.'
>   (Fry, 1954)

References

CADE, S. (1963). Cancer: the patient's viewpoint and the clinician's problems. *Proceedings of the Royal Society of Medicine* **56**, 1.
FEIFEL, H. (Ed.) (1977). Death in contemporary America. In: *New Meanings of Death*, p. 7. McGraw-Hill; New York and Maidenhead.
FRY, C. (1954). *The Dark is Light Enough.* Oxford University Press; London.
HINTON, J. (1963). Mental and physical distress in the dying. *Quarterly Journal of Medicine* **32**, 1.
HINTON, J. (1974). Talking with people about to die. *British Medical Journal* **2**, 25.
HOLFORD, J. M. (1973). *Terminal Care. Care of the dying.* Proceedings of a National Symposium held on 29th November 1972. HMSO; London.
McINTOSH, J. (1977). *Communication and Awareness in a Cancer Ward.* Croom Helm; London. Prodist; New York.
SMITHERS, D. W. (1960). *A Clinical Prospect of the Cancer Problem.* Livingstone; Edinburgh.
SYMINGTON, T. and CARTER, R. L. (Eds.) (1976). Editorial note, p. 673, in *Scientific Foundations of Oncology.* Heinemann Medical; London.
WEISMAN, A. D. (1972). *On Dying and Denying. A psychiatric study of terminality*, p. 93. Behavioral Publications; New York.
WEISMAN, A. D. (1977). The psychiatrist and the inexorable. In: *New Meanings of Death*, pp. 116, 119. Ed. by H. Feifel. McGraw-Hill; New York and Maidenhead.
WEISMAN, A. D. and HACKETT, T. P. (1962). The dying patient. *Forest Hosp. Pub.* **1**, 742.
WITZEL, L. (1975). Behaviour of the dying patient. *British Medical Journal* **2**, 81.

Addenda
I: Editor's Comment on Frontispiece

Few diseases possess the capacity that cancer has to shut a patient off almost completely from those around him. 'It seemed so strange; no-one seemed to want to look at me,' said a patient on admission. When to this emotional isolation physical distress such as constant nausea, intractable dyspnoea or pain are added, a patient may be held a prisoner in a kind of solitary confinement. If to someone trapped in this situation we offer no more than an injection of a narcotic, can we marvel if he becomes drug dependent or asks us for the quick release of death? This does not exaggerate the situation. Here one patient illustrates vividly the feelings of a multitude.

The painting reproduced as the Frontispiece to this book was commissioned from Mr H.Y. when he was an in-patient at St Christopher's Hospice. He had an inoperable squamous cell carcinoma of the bronchus, and summarized histories of his two admissions are given below. Painting was his hobby and, as his condition improved, his bed-table became covered with sketches. We suggested that he might try to illustrate his memory of the pain of his thoracotomy and of a painful acute retention which developed shortly after his admission. The urethritis which had precipitated this was treated successfully; he received one dose of narcotic before he was catheterized and the infection treated with antibiotics. Pain was never a problem for the rest of that admission.

Mr H.Y. depicts his pain surrounding him totally as he lies stretched out on his bed. He described the whorled figures to us as the 'knotted muscles' of tension. He is cut off from the world by it.

This was an acute pain which was treated specifically (Chapters 5 and 6); but the painting could also represent the feelings of many patients with chronic pain for which no specific treatment is available. Too many of them have to endure it or to wait until pain is present before they can expect to be given any relief. 'In our hospital the patients have to earn their morphine' a student reported to us on a hospice ward round. Mr H.Y. painted this picture for us to use as one of our set of slides illustrating the 'total' pain suffered by many patients with terminal disease. There are physical, mental, social and spiritual facets of this whole pain experience, and each calls for our attention. The authors of this book come from their different approaches to give attention to the person who is suffering.

Summary of Mr H.Y.'s First Admission to St Christopher's Hospice

Aged 51   M   Admitted 25/11/70
                               Discharged 27/2/71

Admitted from home, as an emergency at request of general practitioner.

Carcinoma of left bronchus, since July 1970
Bronchoscopy, September 1970;
Thoracotomy, November 1970.

Pain   Has had some pain across thoracic spine and in the scar, but this not his main complaint.

History   July 1970: cough and slight haemoptysis; reported to GP. X-ray then no appreciable disease (NAD). September 1970: repeat x-ray; then bronchoscopy and biopsy showed squamous cell carcinoma of left bronchus. November 1970: thoracotomy; growth found to be inoperable. Sent home after 2 weeks. Appetite poor, vomiting sometimes; dysphagia; marked loss of weight. Sleeps badly; tries to cough but has no strength. Unable to sit up unaided. Very constipated; frequency of micturition. Increasing weakness of both legs. Breathlessness the main problem. Knows that he has a tumour but not the prognosis. Baptist.

On Examination (OE)   Very weak; anaemic; marked signs of breathlessness. Pulse 90. Collapse and consolidation of left chest. Polyneuritis both hands and feet. Parasthesia, loss of feeling and weakness. Very ill and frightened.

Drugs	25/11–27/2	Prednisone	O	5–10 mg t.d.s.
	25/11–27/2	Promazine hydrochloride (Sparine)	O	25 mg t.d.s.
	27/11–27/2	Liver extract (Minamino Compound)		10 ml t.d.s.
	8/12	Diamorphine hydrochloride	O	5 mg s.o.s.
	21/12–24/12	Nitrofurantoin (Furadantin)	O	100 mg q.d.s.
	12/2–27/2	Nitrofurantoin (Furadantin)	O	100 mg q.d.s.

24/12–27/2	Imipramine hydrochloride (Tofranil)	O	25 mg t.d.s.
11/1–3/2	Co-trimoxazole (Septrin)	O	Tabs 2–1 b.d.
3/2–13/2	Sulphomyxin sodium (Thiosporin)	i.m.	500 000 units 6-hourly

Also courses of Chloramphenicol, cloxacillin, nalidixic acid (Negram), dextro-propoxyphene (Distalgesic) from time to time; methagualone hydrochloride (Mandrax) then nitrazepam (Mogadon) at night; chlorpromazine hydrochloride (Largactil) 50 mg at night.

Progress   The acute chest infection was fairly rapidly controlled, patient's appetite improved and he felt better. The polyneuritis slowly resolved and he became ambulant. On 8/12 he developed painful retention requiring catheterization. The urinary infection was resistant but finally improved on Thiosporin. Pain went but frequency remained. Developed a large fluctuant swelling over thoracotomy scar on 1/2/71. This discharged copiously. Patient improved greatly in his general condition, was pain-free, went home for several week-ends and was discharged home on 27/2/71. Will be admitted again if necessary.

Footnote   When Mr H.Y. became acutely ill a few days after his discharge home following his thoracotomy, his family doctor had not received any notification from the hospital. His doctor believed he needed urgent treatment but the hospital had extra beds up and were not able to readmit him.

b.d. = twice a day; i.m. = intramuscular injection; O = oral; q.d.s. = four times a day; s.o.s. = if circumstances require; t.d.s. = three times a day.

Summary of Mr H.Y.'s Second Admission to St Christopher's Hospice

Aged 51   M   Readmitted 3/6/71
Died 14/8/71

Readmitted from the Out-patient Clinic. *See previous summary.*

Carcinoma of left bronchus

Further history   Patient had been discharged home on 27/2/71, since when he had been visited several times and had attended the OP Clinic. He managed very well at first but had repeated chest infections with purulent sputum, treated with antibiotics. Frequency of micturition was troublesome and, on 3/6, patient was complaining of severe pain and was able to pass very little urine each time. For 2 days he had been very sleepy and his mind had been wandering.

Drugs	3/6–12/8	Prednisone	O	10 mg t.d.s.
	3/6–16/6	Promazine hydrochloride (Sparine)	O	25 mg t.d.s.
	11/6–19/6	Co-trimoxazole (Septrin)	O	Tabs 2 b.d.
	9/7–13/7	Co-trimoxazole (Septrin)	O	Tabs 2 b.d.
	20/7–7/8	Co-trimoxazale (Septrin)	O	10 ml b.d.
	16/6–5/7	Diamorphine hydrochloride	O	2·5–5 mg 4-hourly q.d.s.-b.d.-at night
	5/8–14/8	Diamorphine hydrochloride	O/I	2·5–5 mg 4-hourly

16/6–5/7	Prochlorperazine (Stemetil)	O	5 mg 4-hourly-q.d.s.-b.d.-o.d.
3/8–11/8	Prochlorperazine (Stemetil)	O/I	5/6·25–12·5 mg 4-hourly p.r.n.
19/6–10/7	Ampicillin	O	250 mg q.d.s.
23/6–24/7	Diphenhydramine hydrochloride (Benylin)	O	5–10 ml 4-hourly t.d.s.
13/7–20/7	Colistin sulphate (Colomycin)	/I	1 000 000 units t.d.s.
4/8–13/8	Cyclizine	O/I	50/50 mg b.d.

Chlorpromazine hydrochloride (Largactil) 25 mg at night; nitrazepam (Mogadon) 2 tablets at night; methadone linctus 5–10 ml at night p.r.n. hyoscine i.m. 0·4 mg 3 times, 13/8, 14/8.

Progress Catheter passed soon after admission; urine drained well. Remained drowsy and quiet. Cough troublesome and sputum blood-stained. Occasional pain and abdominal distension when catheter became blocked. Bladder wash-outs and catheter changed as needed. Pain controlled by small doses of mist. diamorphine, gradually reduced from 4-hourly to nocte only by 5/7. Became brighter and was pushing himself along in his wheelchair and later walking with a Zimmer walking aid. Took Communion on the ward on 21/7. Not so well by the end of the month, again becoming more drowsy and having episodes of vomiting and nausea. Small doses of regular analgesia restarted. Gradually became weaker, with more frequent vomiting. Remained weak, confused from time to time, but mostly peaceful. Bouts of severe coughing and restlessness at times, which responded to medication. Lapsed into unconsciousness on 13/8, remained very peaceful and died at 00.35 hours on 14/8/71.

Footnote His wife wrote after his death about the extra 8 months of his life that the whole family had enjoyed. They still keep in touch with the Hospice.

b.d. = twice a day; i.m. = intramuscular injection; O = oral; O/I = oral/injection; I = injection; o.d. = once a day; p.r.n. = as the occasion arises; q.d.s. = four times a day; t.d.s. = three times a day

II. Facts and Figures

B. Joan Haram

Editorial note
Many of the chapters of this book come from the background of the work of St Christopher's Hospice, which admits over 600 patients a year—the great majority of them suffering from terminal cancer. It was our policy from the beginning to add to controlled clinical trials of narcotics (Chapter 5) and psychosocial studies, the careful monitoring of our daily clinical experience by maintaining a system of records from which we could retrieve the maximum of information. The following description of Dr Haram's work illustrates our good fortune in having had one Recorder for the past ten years.

Some statistics drawn from our analysed and detailed records, and a record of the control of pain sustained during one year, are included below. These records have been an invaluable resource to Dr Twycross and Dr Parkes in their work and to the developing clinical experience of the Hospice. It is hoped that it will also be a resource for others in the future.

The Clinical Studies team includes a self-styled 'Recorder' whose work is to compose a summary of each patient's case notes, if possible from the onset of symptoms until discharge or death. In a little under ten years, between 24th July 1967 when the Hospice opened and 15th May 1977, 5000 such summaries have been compiled. Each is fitted to a Cope-Chat punch card * from which over 250 items of information can be extracted and analysed for statistical purposes and research. A copy is retained in the notes, another copy is sent to the hospital or doctor previously attended by the patient.

The basic format of the summary has remained unchanged, the content becoming increasingly succinct and additional details being incorporated as the work of the Hospice expanded. Data include history of illness, diagnosis, treatment, present symptoms, mobility, insight, home circumstances, reason for admission and whether this has been from hospital or home. If the patient has been under the care of the domiciliary service of the Hospice, this is reported. Pain, being of special significance, is mentioned under a separate heading. All this material is culled from various sources, such as doctors' letters, nurses' notes and hospital reports. Examination by the doctor admitting the patient to the Hospice follows. Drugs prescribed are listed, with dates of starting and stopping each drug, increased dosages given, and, when possible, any change from oral to parenteral administration. The progress of the illness is described and, if the patient remains at St Christopher's Hospice for any length of time, particular events are noted. These would include visits home, further treatment, insight during stay and unexpected developments. If death occurs, the terminal symptoms and mode of dying are recorded.

The summaries provide a simple basis for monitoring and modifying clinical results. For example, the number of patients within a given period who received 60 mg or more of diamorphine four-hourly have been studied and the effects of the treatment assessed; notes of patients admitted between July 1967 and June 1976 with squamous cell carcinomas of the head and neck are at present being reviewed. The use of anti-inflammatory drugs in the control of bone pain is being monitored and other studies are planned.

Some representative data, based on the records of St Christopher's Hospice, are shown in Figs. 1.3–1.5 and in Tables 1.1–1.4.

---

* Paramount card by Copeland Chatterson Co. Ltd.

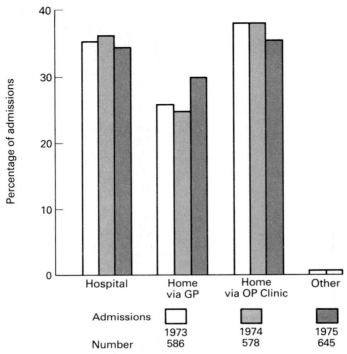

Fig. 1.3. Breakdown of admissions to St Christopher's Hospice: from another hospital, from home via the general practitioner, from home via the Hospice Out-patient Clinic, and from elsewhere, 1973–1975 inclusive.

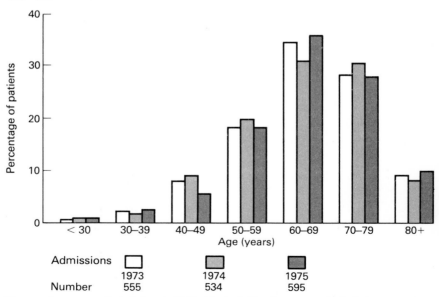

Fig. 1.4. Age groups of admissions to St Christopher's Hospice, 1973–1975 inclusive.

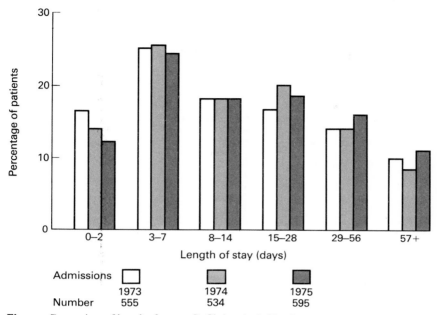

Fig. 1.5. Comparison of length of stay at St Christopher's Hospice, 1973–1975 inclusive.

Table 1.1   Primary site of malignant tumour (grouped): admissions to St Christopher's Hospice, 1974–1976

	1976 (%)	1975 (%)	1974 (%)
Gastrointestinal tract	24·75	25·75	25·0
Bronchus	21·5	23·5	22·0
Breast	18·25	17·0	16·0
Genitourinary tract	15·0	12·25	16·5
Central nervous system	4·25	3·5	4·5
Head and neck	3·0	3·0	4·0
Pancreas	2·75	4·25	4·5
Sarcomas (various sites)	1·75	2·5	0·5
Melanoma (various sites)	1·25	1·25	2·0
Miscellaneous	1·0	1·5	1·0
Unknown	6·5	5·5	4·0

Figures rounded off to nearest 0·25 per cent.

Table 1.2 Pain statistics, St Christopher's Hospice 1976
A. *Pain was not a problem in 206 (34%) of patients on admission*

Source of referral	Male	Female	Total
Other hospital	35	46	81
Via GP	38	28	66
Via OP Clinic	31	28	59
Total	104	102	206

14 of these patients subsequently complained of pain; all had good relief

B. *Pain was a problem in 401 (66%) of patients on admission*

Admitted from	Male	Female	Total
Other hospital	44	96	140
Via GP	69	66	135
Via OP Clinic	54	72	126
Total	167	234	401

All but 10 patients obtained good relief from pain:
  details of 6 patients whose pain was difficult to control are given in Table 1.3
  3 patients died within 1 day
  1 died within 2 days of admission (appeared to have pain on movement)
  1 patient (carcinoma right breast) with an oedematous arm needed extra analgesia before
  painful dressing was attempted.

Table 1.3 Details of patients whose pain was difficult to control (Table 1.2B)

	Sex/Age	Primary site	Survival (days)	Details
1.	F/52	Carcinomas, left and right breasts	51	On admission, severe pain in lumbar region. Had been having diamorphine 65 mg 4-hourly. Cheerful but pain severe at times between drug rounds. Nerve block considered unsuitable. Lost all sensation in legs. Discomfort continued but usually had good nights. Intermittent pain was more difficult to control during last 7–10 days. Enjoyed going to a choral recital 3 days prior to peaceful death. O/IM diamorphine 60–80 mg 4-hourly. Phenylbutazone (Butacote) 100–200 mg t.d.s.–q.d.s.
2.	F/40	Carcinoma, right breast	14 & 7	Pain in head, neck and spine. Brave but tense. Young family, five sons aged 4–13. Knew diagnosis and believed pain would go because of radiotherapy. Became pain-free on O diamorphine 5 mg 4-hourly and phenylbutazone (Butacote) 200 mg t.d.s. dothiepin (Prothiaden) 25 mg t.d.s. Discharged home. Readmitted after 7 weeks with acute pain in neck which occurred as she was lifting turkey from the oven. Pain radiated up both sides of head and restricted neck movement. Neck numb which worried her but she became more relaxed and cheerful. X-ray showed pathological fracture at

Sex/Age	Primary site	Survival (days)	Details
			C2. Knew about fracture, was frightened but was reassured and became peaceful. Given cervical collar. Developed broncho-pneumonia—coughing aggravated pain. Deteriorated rapidly, became unconscious and died peacefully. Diamorphine increased to O/I 10–20 mg 4-hourly.
3. F/48	Carcinoma, left upper lobe bronchus	43	History of severe pain prior to admission; almost bent double in attempt to get relief. Had been taking methadone 'apparently in vast quantities with little regard for amount or time'. Husband had left her to live with another woman 4 months before admission. She settled in well, appeared bright but was labile. Pain continued to be a problem when moving her despite increasing analgesia. Pain also varied considerably on account of social and emotional problems. Peaceful death. Had dothiepin (Prothiaden) 25 mg b.d., dextropropoxyphene (Distalgesic) 2 tablets p.r.n., O/I diamorphine 30–90 mg 4-hourly.
4. F/47	Carcinoma, left breast	43	Pain, which was partly controlled by diamorphine 35 mg 3-hourly before admission, in back, groin and lower abdomen. Tearful and depressed. Settled well but pain needed increasing analgesia. Anxious to go home to Jamaica but eventually realized she was not going to get better and was happy to stay. At this time pain no longer a problem. Drugs included diazepam (Valium), prochlorperazine (Stemetil) dihydrocodeine tartrate (DF 118) and dextropropoxyphene (Distalgesic), O/I diamorphine 30–60 mg 4-hourly.
5. M/38	Chondrosarcoma of sacrum	13	History of 4 years of pain before admission. In for 2 months in 1975. After pain was controlled he went home for 3 weeks, during which time he was almost pain-free. Readmitted for reassessment. Weak and depressed but still hoped to go home again. Pain not always fully controlled, seemed ready for his drugs. Social problems; often very depressed. Sudden deterioration before peaceful death. Phenylbutazone (Butacote) 100–200 mg q.d.s.–t.d.s. O/I diamorphine 40/30 mg 4-hourly.
6. M/56	Carcinoma, left bronchus	12	Pain left hip, thigh, knee and leg. Emaciated at admission. Analgesia increased but pain remained difficult to control. Alternate nights appeared to be fairly comfortable. Anxious about finances and seen by Medical Social Worker. Died peacefully. Dextropropoxyphene (Distalgesic) p.r.n. O/I diamorphine 10–30 mg 4-hourly.

b.d. = twice a day; O/I = oral to injection; p.r.n. = as the occasion arose; q.d.s. = four times a day; t.d.s. = three times a day.

Table 1.4   Analgesics, St Christopher's Hospice 1976

A. Of 607 patients with malignant disease, 33 (5·5%) received no diamorphine: 8 of these (3 males and 5 females) received another analgesic 'as required', and 20 received no analgesic.

The pain experienced by the other 5 was satisfactorily controlled on

Drug	Male	Female	Total
Dextropropoxyphene (Distalgesic)	—	3	3
Dipipanone and cyclizine (Diconal)	1	—	1
Pentazocine hydrochloride (Fortral)	1	—	1

52 (8·6%) patients (19 males and 33 females) had phenylbutazone.   Almost all patients had a phenothiazine.

74 (12·2%) patients (24 males and 50 females) had a tricyclic antidepressant.

252 (41·5%) patients (105 males and 147 females) had diazepam.

574 (94·6%) patients received diamorphine at some time during their stay.

B. *Maximum individual dose of diamorphine as prescribed either orally or by injection*

Individual dose (mg)	Male	Female	Total	%	Cumulative %
2·5	29	42	71	12·25	12·25
5	62	69	131	22·75	35·00
10	71	65	136	23·75	58·75
15	21	32	53	9·25	68·00
20	29	48	77	13·50	81·50
30	26	23	49	8·50	90·00
40	13	21	34	6·00	96·00
60	4	10	14	2·50	98·50
Over 60	3	6	9	1·50	100·00
Total	258	316	574	100·00	

Percentages rounded off to nearest 0·25 per cent.

2

Pathological Aspects

R. L. Carter

Editorial Note

'Finally, the physician should bear in mind that he himself is not exempt from the common lot, but subject to the same laws of mortality and disease as others, and he will care for the sick with more diligence and tenderness if he remembers that he himself is their fellow sufferer.'

(Sydenham, 1666)

Sydenham asked for diligence, tenderness and the recognition of human fellowship. Nowhere are these more needed than for those who are suffering from mortal illness.

'Diligence' could sum up many of the chapters of this book which begins with a discussion of the pathological and physical processes underlying the problems of those with terminal malignant disease. It must involve the ever more assiduous search for the causes that lie behind symptoms, their treatment, and the complex nature of terminal pain, almost an illness in itself. It means learning the details of current methods of pain control, but it also means looking towards new knowledge of its mechanisms and possible further treatment. It means the discriminating use of radiotherapy so that the minimum amount of time is spent waiting and travelling and the maximum at home, with few symptoms to contend with over and above those already present from the disease process. It means the balancing of cytotoxic drugs to the needs of each individual patient and the balancing of time spent in hospital after surgery against time spent at home—the place where most people wish to spend their last days.

Diligence means care for choices, efficiency, persistent imagination and responsible decision-making. It could be the one word which sums up a great part of this book.

But tenderness means awareness of common humanity and recognition of the person who is ill, allowing him choices and options—sometimes where they seem irrational and even irresponsible—understanding where someone chooses to be for his last weeks, and how he plans to help those he leaves.

Reference

SYDENHAM, Thomas London (1666). *Methodus Curandi Febres.*

'But who could tell? Even doctors, how could they detect whether the solitary, destructive cells had or hadn't stolen through the darkness like landing craft, and where they had anchored?'
(Solzhenitsyn, 1968)

Advanced malignant disease presents diverse and often complex problems in diagnosis and clinical management. A preliminary description of the underlying pathology is therefore necessary to provide a context in which such problems can be viewed.

A schematic and highly simplified representation of certain aspects of the natural history of progressive tumour growth is shown in Fig. 2.1. Three somewhat arbitrary phases may be recognized: subclinical disease; clinically early disease; clinically advanced disease. The first phase is illustrated by a tumour comprising approximately 10^9 cells and weighing about 1 g. Unless superficially located, such a lesion will *not* be detectable clinically; it will only be revealed by appropriate cancer screening tests if such are available. The tumour is likely to be localized, but invasion and metastasis may have begun. Clinically early disease usually corresponds to a tumour of approximately 2×10^9 cells. An unknown proportion of patients will already have occult metastases, their numbers and location varying according to the type of tumour. Most patients present at this stage. The third phase—clinically advanced disease—is the theme of this chapter: the patient will by now have widespread disease with perhaps a total burden of tumour amounting to about 10^{12} cells, representing 1 kg of tumour tissue. The semiquantitative approach adopted here serves to emphasize the sheer mass of tumour which may be

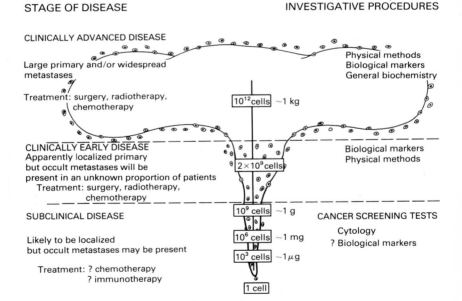

STAGE OF DISEASE   INVESTIGATIVE PROCEDURES

CLINICALLY ADVANCED DISEASE

Large primary and/or widespread
metastases   Physical methods
                                                    Biological markers
                                                    General biochemistry
Treatment: surgery, radiotherapy,
        chemotherapy 10^{12}cells ~1 kg

CLINICALLY EARLY DISEASE
Apparently localized primary   Biological markers
but occult metastases will be   Physical methods
present in an unknown proportion of patients 2×10^9cells
    Treatment: surgery, radiotherapy,
            chemotherapy

SUBCLINICAL DISEASE 10^9 cells ~1 g   CANCER SCREENING TESTS

                                                        Cytology
Likely to be localized 10^6 cells ~1 mg   ? Biological markers
but occult metastases may be present
                                    10^3 cells ~1 μg
    Treatment: ? chemotherapy
             ? immunotherapy
                                    1 cell

Fig. 2.1. Some aspects of the natural history of progressive tumour growth. The three (arbitrary) stages of disease are illustrated, together with general comments on appropriate methods of investigation and clinical management. The scheme is selective and over-simplified, omitting important considerations such as fluctuations in the rate of tumour cell proliferation, tumour cell loss and effects of treatment. The approximate weights of the lesions (~1 μg, ~1 mg, ~1 g) take no account of the non-neoplastic supporting stroma. (Reproduced, with permission, from Symington and Carter, 1976.)

present. This, in turn, throws some light on the progressive failure of radical surgery, radiotherapy and chemotherapy; it provides a rationale for the eventual change of tactics from control of disease to control of symptoms and palliation; and it gives at least an indication of the complexities of advanced malignant disease which need further investigation.

The Primary Tumour

In most patients the primary tumour will have been previously treated. There is often no evidence of any residual primary neoplasm, and the patient presents with disseminated disease. In certain circumstances, however, the primary tumour may still be present though almost always accompanied by metastases:

1. The lesion may have been neglected and the patient has delayed seeking medical advice. Such cases, often presenting as large fungating masses, are sometimes encountered in breast, cervix, vulva and skin.

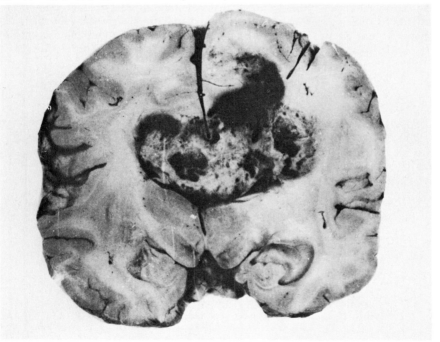

Fig. 2.2. Glioblastoma multiforme—a highly aggressive tumour which grows rapidly and infiltrates the surrounding brain substance. This tumour arose in the right parietal lobe and has spread across the midline, destroying the corpus callosum, blocking and distorting the lateral ventricles and invading the opposite cerebral hemisphere. The right cerebrum is markedly swollen, and there is extensive haemorrhage in and around the tumour. The clinical picture accompanying a tumour of this kind can be readily inferred, with symptoms and signs initially referable to the right parietal lobe, becoming more diffuse as the tumour spreads within the brain substance and blocks the lateral ventricles. This, combined with the associated haemorrhage and oedema, results in a progressive increase in intracranial pressure.

2. Primary tumours may be refractory to treatment or, more frequently, they recur after treatment. Local recurrences, which can usually be regarded as one manifestation of more generalized metastatic disease, are most often seen in cancers of the breast and of the head and neck, less frequently at the sites of surgical scars, stomata, fistulae, amputation stumps, and in peripherally arising melanomas and sarcomas of soft tissues and bone. Local recurrences vary in size and appearance; multiple 'satellite' lesions may occur. Local recurrence is virtually certain if the tumour has not been completely ablated. This situation is illustrated by gliomas infiltrating vital or inaccessible parts of the brain and spinal cord. Systemic metastases from primary tumours of the central nervous system are excessively rare, and patients die with *local* infiltrative disease (Fig. 2.2).

3. The primary tumour may be minute and elude detection. Despite its size, such a tumour can metastasize widely and 'carcinomatosis, primary unknown' is a familiar problem in clinical oncology. Certain sites for minute primary tumours fall under particular suspicion in such circumstances—breast, bronchus, thyroid, testis and, occasionally, stomach and kidney. Efforts should be made to localize these elusive primary lesions, despite the presence of advanced disease, as such information may modify the overall clinical management. But the problem often remains and, even after a meticulous autopsy, the pathologist is sometimes unable to determine the primary focus of disease.

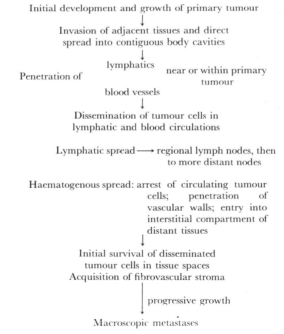

Fig. 2.3. A simplified scheme of the metastatic process. The emphasis here is on lymphatic and vascular spread, but several other, less important, modes of tumour dissemination also operate. The scheme emphasizes that metastasis comprises a sequence of interlocking processes, sometimes referred to as the metastatic 'cascade'. (Reproduced, with permission, from Symington and Carter, 1976.)

Metastatic Tumours

Most of the common fatal tumours kill because they metastasize; rarely is death directly attributable to the primary lesion itself. Metastasis is a complex and ill-understood process, the basic elements of which are summarized in Fig. 2.3.

The common sites of metastatic tumour (with particular reference to carcinomas) are illustrated in Fig. 2.4, and some of these are discussed briefly below.

Lymph nodes

Most carcinomas, and some melanomas and neuroblastomas, spread initially via the local lymphatic vessels to the nearest group of lymph nodes. The lymphatics are invaded by tumour cells either singly or in clumps; if the process is massive and accompanied by a measure of local lymphatic obstruction, it can sometimes be observed clinically—for example, in superficial malignant melanomas, and in breast cancer with its 'peau d'orange' effect.

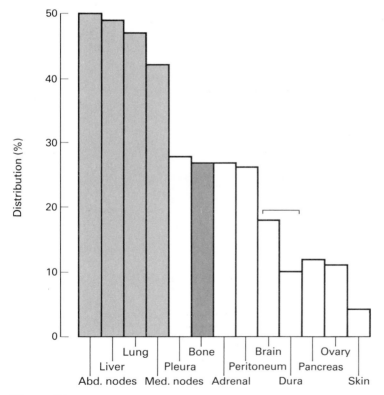

Fig. 2.4. Distribution of macroscopic metastases in 1000 consecutive autopsies on patients with carcinoma of various sites. The study was made at the Montefiore Hospital for Chronic Diseases, New York. The principal sites for metastatic tumour are intra-abdominal and mediastinal lymph nodes, liver, lungs and pleura, and bone. (Based on data from Abrams, Spiro and Goldstein, 1950.)

Once established in the regional lymph nodes, the tumour cells grow and replace the normal nodal structures. Afferent lymph flow is progressively distorted and incoming tumour cells are deflected to fresh lymph nodes in contiguous anatomical groups. In most instances, lymph node involvement follows a fairly orderly pattern which is broadly predictable on anatomical grounds (Fig. 2.5). Lymph nodes replaced by metastatic tumour are usually enlarged, sometimes greatly so, and can cause symptoms and signs as a result of pressure on or erosion into adjacent structures. Large superficial lymph node metastases—in the neck, axillae, groins—occasionally ulcerate through the skin.

Lymph node metastases must be distinguished from enlarged lymph nodes due to primary malignancies of the lymphoid system—Hodgkin's disease and

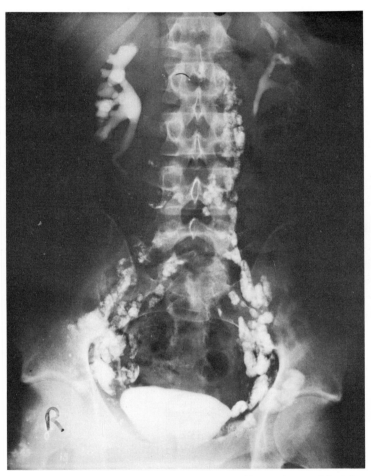

Fig. 2.5. Lymphangiogram from a 25-year-old man with a seminoma of the left testis. The tumour has metastasized to the pelvic and para-aortic nodes and, on the right side, there is compression and kinking of the ureter which is giving rise to a hydronephrosis. Despite this extensive intra-abdominal metastatic disease, the tumour regressed in response to radiotherapy and chemotherapy. The patient remains well 4 years later.

the non-Hodgkin's lymphomas. This group of neoplasms is usually multifocal in origin, involving some or all of the lymphoid system together with a variable degree of spread to non-lymphoid structures such as liver, bone marrow, gut, soft tissues and skin. Enlarged lymph nodes may also be encountered in the leukaemias.

Liver

The liver is a major site for metastases from intra-abdominal malignancies, particularly carcinomas of the colon and rectum, stomach and pancreas. The main route of access is via the radicles of the hepatic portal venous system. Blood- (or lymph-) borne hepatic metastases may also be derived from primary cancers of the breast and lungs. Haematogenous spread to the liver, with sometimes massive involvement, is common in disseminating malignant melanoma (Fig. 2.6).

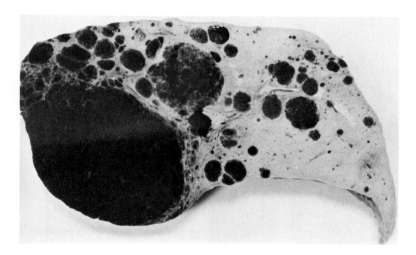

Fig. 2.6. Liver metastases. The patient, a woman of 44, developed malignant melanoma in the right eye. The orbit was cleared and she remained well for 10 years. Her liver then became tender and enlarged rapidly, and she lost weight, developed several pigmented skin nodules, and became increasingly breathless and confused. At autopsy she was found to have widespread malignant melanoma with metastases in the brain, lungs and pleura, pericardium, liver, lymph nodes, kidneys, peritoneum, bones and skin. The liver was enormously enlarged, weighing 9·5 kg; the Figure shows the cut surface with numerous deposits of heavily pigmented metastatic melanoma.

Intrahepatic metastases are generally numerous and sometimes very large; haemorrhage and necrosis are often marked. The whole organ, studded with deposits, may fill the abdomen and weigh several kilograms. The clinical findings of a large, palpable liver, often tender and with a knobbly edge, are easy to interpret. Jaundice may be due to intrahepatic metastases or, less often, to extrinsic biliary obstruction as a result of lymph node metastases in the porta hepatis.

Lungs

Most pulmonary metastases (Fig. 2.7) are derived from tumour cells which invade peripheral capillaries and venules in the systemic circulation. Sarcomas, in particular, metastasize to the lungs in the blood-stream; so, too, do several carcinomas, though these also reach the lungs via lymphatics—for example, from the breast. The overlying pleura is frequently involved, and

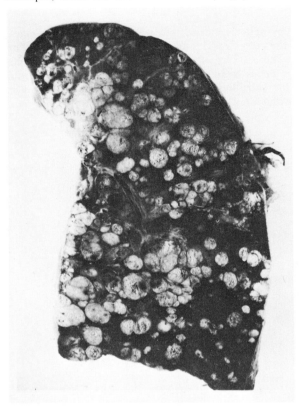

Fig. 2.7. Lung metastases. The patient, a boy of 14, developed an osteosarcoma in the right femur. The leg was disarticulated at the hip and he received chemotherapy. Multiple lung metastases appeared at 16 months and grew rapidly. At autopsy, metastatic disease was confined to the lungs and the Figure illustrates massive pulmonary involvement by secondary osteosarcoma. The small amount of uninvolved lung substance is dark as a result of intrapulmonary congestion and haemorrhage.

pleural effusions are a common clinical concomitant (see later). Intrapulmonary metastases are usually multiple and vary in size, the larger lesions tending to become haemorrhagic. They are associated with varying degrees of local oedema, congestion, haemorrhage and infection in the uninvolved parenchyma. Large deposits may obstruct peripheral bronchi and bronchioles; obstruction of major bronchi is usually due to enlarged mediastinal lymph nodes. Varying degrees of atelectasis, with or without infection, will result. As in the liver, there may be progressive loss of normal function, with death ensuing from organ failure (cf. Fig. 2.9).

Bones

Skeletal metastases are almost always blood-borne; direct invasion of bone is uncommon except with certain squamous cell carcinomas—for example, bronchus, tongue and oral cavity, cervix uteri. Some primary cancers show a particular predilection to metastasize to bone (breast, prostate, kidney, thyroid, lung) and to involve particular sites. The axial skeleton (skull, ribs and sternum, vertebrae, pelvis, upper humerus and femur) is frequently infiltrated while more peripheral bones, lacking marrow cavities, are usually free of metastatic tumour (Fig. 2.8).

Once established within the skeleton, tumour cells evoke complex local reactions of bone destruction and new bone formation; the marrow cavities are invaded to the extent that tumour cells can be identified in bone marrow aspiration; and extensive destruction of bone may result in pathological fractures and compression of adjacent structures such as the spinal cord and nerve roots. Hypercalcaemia may occur but this change, which is also encountered in cancer patients without overt bone metastases, may also reflect ectopic hormone production by the tumour (see later; also Chapter 3).

Body cavities

Invasion of the peritoneal, pleural and pericardial cavities by disseminating tumour is common in advanced malignant disease. It is usually a result of direct spread, either from the primary tumour itself or from adjacent metastases. Serosal deposits are generally multiple and tend to 'seed' throughout the involved cavity. They are frequently accompanied by effusions of protein-rich, blood-stained fluid in which tumour cells can be identified. Many litres of fluid may accumulate in the peritoneal and pleural cavity, producing intense abdominal discomfort and dyspnoea. Secondary infection may supervene, particularly in the pleura. Repeated paracenteses tend to induce fibrosis, with loculation of fluid. Peritoneal effusions (ascites, carcinomatosis peritonei) are most often associated with carcinomas of the ovary and, to a lesser extent, stomach, large bowel and pancreas; pleural effusions with carcinomas of breast, lung and oesophagus and with pulmonary metastases from various sources. These same three primary tumours may also induce pericardial effusions resulting in low-grade pericarditis or fatal cardiac tamponade. Some intracranial tumours, notably medulloblastomas and ependymomas, occasionally seed along the spaces surrounding the neuraxis.

Some of the basic patterns of cancer dissemination have been described, and certain qualifying comments about metastasis must now be added.

1. It is a clinical commonplace that malignant tumours vary in their capacity to metastasize. It was noted earlier that gliomas kill by invading locally within the central nervous system, and that distant metastases are almost unknown (see Fig. 2.2). Other tumours—testicular teratomas, some melanomas, 'oat-cell' carcinomas of the bronchus—tend to disseminate exceptionally widely.

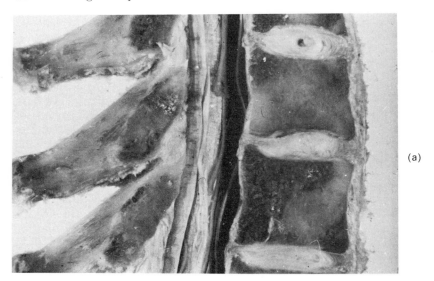

(a)

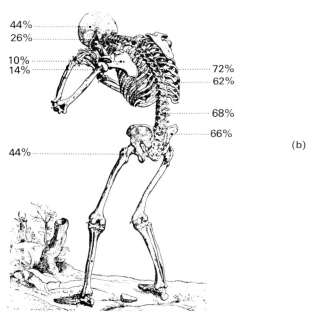

44%
26%

10%
14%

72%
62%

68%

66%

44%

(b)

Fig. 2.8. Bone metastases (a) Vertebral bodies infiltrated by metastasizing carcinoma of the breast. The tumour is replacing much of the marrow spaces and bone trabeculae but the cartilaginous intervertebral discs and the periosteum are not involved. There is no evidence of extension into the spinal canal here, but compression of the cord and/or nerve roots may complicate metastatic disease in the spine. (b) The distribution of bone metastases in carcinoma of the breast. The skeleton is from Vesalius' *De Humani Corporis Fabrica* of 1543; the superimposed figures, which show the distribution of skeletal deposits detected by scintigraphy in 50 patients, are quoted from Galasko (1972).

The basis for this spectrum of 'metastatic potential' in different malignant tumours is unknown, but it is crucial to the understanding of the metastatic process.

2. The number, size and distribution of metastatic tumours all vary, a point made clear by two of the preceding illustrations. Malignant melanoma (see Fig. 2.6) and osteosarcoma (see Fig. 2.7) are both tumours with a high metastatic potential and both the examples quoted had metastasized, mainly by the blood-stream; but the malignant melanoma produced massive disease in many sites whereas the osteosarcoma spread to the lungs but apparently nowhere else. Again, the amount of tumour present may vary enormously for a given neoplasm. In carcinomas of the breast or bronchus, for example, one patient may have solitary or a few scattered deposits while another is riddled with metastases equivalent to perhaps 1 kg or more of tumour tissue (see Fig. 2.1). It is essential to stress that the distribution of metastases is non-random, and that there are definite sites of predilection. It was made clear in Fig. 2.4 that certain tissues and organs are regularly involved by metastases; equally, certain primary tumours appear to metastasize preferentially to particular sites. Breast cancers, for example, frequently involve the adrenals and ovaries; 'oat-cell' carcinomas of the bronchus also show a high incidence of adrenal metastases. (Both adrenal and ovarian metastases are likely to be clinically occult.) Conversely, other sites are rarely involved. There is no mention in Fig. 2.4 of the heart, spleen or skeletal muscle: although these structures have a rich blood supply and, in the case of skeletal muscle, comprise a large proportion of the total body mass, involvement by metastatic tumour is uncommon.

3. Previous mention of occult adrenal and ovarian metastases emphasizes the important point that a proportion of metastatic disease in any one patient almost always goes undetected during life. Clinical findings, alone, are imprecise and more accurate appraisal of tumour spread can be made by additional investigations as diverse as radiology (including scintigraphy, arteriography, lymphangiography and computerized axial tomography), isotope and ultrasonic scans, serum enzyme level estimations, bone marrow aspiration, tissue biopsy and surgical staging procedures. Despite these techniques, however, the detection of metastatic disease remains a major problem in clinical oncology; and, in general, most clinicians tend to underestimate the amount and extent of metastatic tumour which is eventually found at autopsy.

4. There is mounting evidence that metastases at different sites in the same patient may grow at different rates and differ in their response to irradiation or to chemotherapy. In breast cancer, for example, bone metastases sometimes respond to treatment while soft tissue deposits continue to grow. Metastatic growth is almost always progressive; exceptionally, the tempo of the disease declines and a partial or even complete remission sets in. Such remissions are almost always temporary, and their rarity is stressed.

5. The assumption of an orderly progression of malignant disease—with an overt primary tumour followed after a while by metastases—is fallacious. Several variant patterns may be encountered. The disease may first declare itself by metastatic rather than primary tumour—unexplained anaemia, lymphadenopathy, a pathological fracture—while the primary lesion remains occult. The interval between recognition of a primary tumour and the development of metastases is also variable and, with many tumours, clinical exper-

ience indicates that the metastatic process is often under way by the time the patient first presents with an ostensibly localized lesion. On the other hand, many years may elapse before metastases become apparent, as in some carcinomas of the breast and kidney and malignant melanoma (see Fig. 2.6). The reasons for these long-protracted latent periods—perhaps 15 or 20 years—are wholly obscure.

General Aspects of Advanced Malignant Disease: The Role of Modern Pathology

The effects of disseminated tumour are now recognized to be both complex and subtle. Certain complications of extensive tumour growth have long been familiar, such as pressure on and distortion of normal structures resulting in obstruction, fistula formation, haemorrhage, ulceration and infection. Some of these local effects may have more extensive consequences: compression of the ureters, for example, may result in hydronephrosis (see Fig. 2.5) and progressive loss of functional renal parenchyma. More recently, an increasing number of effects, local and systemic, attributable to products synthesized and released by tumour cells, have been described. The tumour products include a wide variety of 'ectopic' hormones, oncofetal antigens and pharmacological agents such as prostaglandins and tumour angiogenesis factor; their local targets include bone and blood vessels; and their (remote) systematic effects include metabolic derangements (cachexia, abnormal purine metabolism, hyperglycaemia, hypercalcaemia), fever, autoimmune disorders, deranged immune function, and disturbances in the skin, joints and nervous system. Some of these topics are discussed in Chapter 3, but they are noted here to emphasize the scope of modern pathology and the need for modern pathological techniques to be deployed in investigating some of the complexities of advanced malignant disease. It cannot, however, be stressed too strongly that any such investigations must be clearly directed towards the needs of the patient and must never involve him in discomfort, distress or exertion.

One, more traditional, role of the pathologist should finally be noted. Patients with advanced malignant disease often present unexplained features during life; and their precise mode of death is frequently unclear. Information which could be deployed in the practical management of future cases is needlessly lost by a reluctance to request or perform autopsies on such patients. The pathologist can determine the extent of disease reasonably accurately, specific problems in clinical management can sometimes be clarified, and more precise causes of death established (Fig. 2.9). Infections (particularly by gram-negative bacteria and by 'opportunistic' organisms), massive extension into vital organs, and haemorrhage are usually easy to demonstrate; the patients dying with 'carcinomatosis' who lack an obvious specific cause of death are more challenging. An autopsy also provides an unrivalled opportunity to examine the consequences of radiotherapy and chemotherapy and to evaluate effects on vital parenchymatous organs. With the increasing use of complex chemotherapy schedules, such information is urgently needed. Limited post-mortem examinations, directed to a particular clinical question, can be invaluable and involve negligible time and facilities.

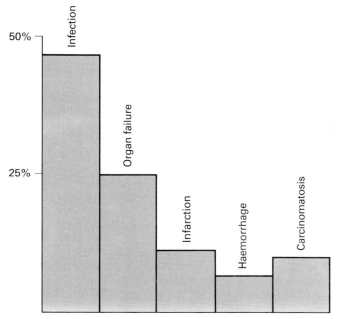

Fig. 2.9. Causes of death in 816 cancer patients at the M. D. Anderson Hospital, Tumor Institute, Houston, Texas. All patients had a complete autopsy.

Notes

Infections. Mostly septicaemia and/or major visceral infections such as pneumonia, peritonitis or pyelonephritis; gram-negative bacteria (*Escherichia coli*, Klebsiella spp., *Pseudomonas aeruginosa*) predominate.

Organ failure. Lungs > heart > liver > CNS > kidneys; mainly or exclusively the consequence of tumour invasion except for cardiac insufficiency.

Infarction. Lungs > heart; pulmonary emboli derived about equally from distal venous thrombosis and from tumour cells.

Haemorrhage. Gastrointestinal tract > brain > ruptured vessel > lungs; Related to underlying tumour and/or to thrombocytopenia or other bleeding diathesis.

Carcinomatosis. Usually severe emaciation and/or electrolyte abnormalities with extensive disseminating disease but no other specific pathological process.

Several patients will have one or more of these 'causes' of death — for example, a combination of infection and organ failure. The incidence of the various causes will in part reflect selection of patients. Fatal haemorrhage due to thrombocytopenia will be more common in units with a special interest in leukaemias and lymphomas. (Based on data from Inagaki, Rodriguez and Bodey, 1974.)

Acknowledgements

I am indebted to the clinicians of the Royal Marsden Hospital for permission to quote details of cases under their care; also to the staff of the Photographic Department for preparing the illustrations.

References and further reading

ABRAMS, H. L., SPIRO, R. and GOLDSTEIN, N. (1950). *Cancer, N.Y.* **3**, 74.

BALDWIN, R. W. (Ed.) (1978). *Secondary Spread of Cancer.* Academic Press, London and New York.

BECKER, F. F. (Ed.) (1975). *Cancer, a comprehensive treatise,* Vols. 1–4. Plenum Press; New York and London.

GALASKO, C. S. B. (1972). *Annals of the Royal College of Surgeons of England* **50**, 3.

HOLLAND, J. F. and FREI, E. (1973). *Cancer Medicine.* Lea & Febiger; Philadelphia.

INAGAKI, J., RODRIGUEZ, V. and BODEY, G. P. (1974). *Cancer, Philadelphia* **33**, 568.

KLASTERSKY, J., DANEAU, D. and VERHEST, A. (1972). *European Journal of Cancer* **8**, 149.

SOLZHENITSYN, A. (1968). *Cancer Ward,* part II. Bodley Head; London.

SYMINGTON, T. and CARTER, R. L. (Eds.) (1976). *Scientific Foundations of Oncology.* Heinemann Medical; London.

WILLIS, R. A. (1973). *The Spread of Tumours in the Human Body,* 3rd edn. Butterworths; London.

3

Physical Aspects
K. C. Calman

'I am not so much afraid of death as ashamed thereof

Sir Thomas Browne

'Protect me
From a body without death. Such indignity
Would be outcast, like a rock in the sea.
But with death, it can hold
More than time gives it, or the earth shows it.'
Fry, 1954

Terminal illness in cancer patients occurs when such patients have been accurately diagnosed, in whom death does not seem far off and in whom medical effort has turned from the curative to the palliative. This definition carries three implications:

1. That the diagnosis has been firmly established, and that the symptoms and signs present are related to progressive malignant disease and not primarily to conditions which are not terminal;
2. That it is possible to give some prediction of the time of death;
3. That conventional anticancer therapy has been used to the full.

What are the main symptoms and signs?

Both should emerge from a careful clinical history and examination, the importance of which cannot be over-emphasized.

The history

Close attention must be paid to the clinical history. Only when a patient's problems have been adequately described (and understood) can there be a rational approach to treatment. Traditionally, the clinical history is pieced together in a system-by-system enquiry; but while this has the merit of thoroughness it is often more useful to adopt a problem-orientated approach with the terminally ill patient. Each symptom—pain, nausea, breathlessness—is described and, after examination, a clinical diagnosis made. The various findings are then collated, specific investigations are undertaken where necessary and treatment is arranged. The response to treatment is carefully documented and any subsequent modifications necessary for more effective symptom control are made.

Certain specific questions should be asked, including the following.

Pain. Site, severity, time and time-intensity relationships? What makes it better or worse? The management of pain is fully discussed in Chapter 5; the more information available, the easier it should be to determine the underlying aetiology and begin appropriate pain-controlling measures.

Mouth problems. Ulcers, soreness, dysphagia, thirst, changes in taste?

Appetite. The amount and type of food taken? Does anorexia occur at the thought of food? Does anything alleviate this anorexia?

Nausea and vomiting. When does it occur? What provokes or improves it?

Breathlessness. Provoking causes, particularly in relation to movement and posture? Time relationships? Associations with cough? What makes it better or worse?

Episodes of bleeding. Haemoptysis, haematemesis and melaena, haematuria, vaginal and rectal bleeding?

Disturbances in bowel and bladder functions. Incontinence, dysuria, discharges? Are surgical stomata functioning adequately?

Sleeplessness. What, in particular, are its time relationships? Is it linked to pain or breathlessness or urinary frequency?

The quantification of symptoms, though difficult, is often useful in the assessment of treatment. Symptoms such as pain, anorexia or vomiting may be scored as mild, moderate or severe, or by a series of pluses: $-$, $+$, $++$, $+++$. Alternatively, a linear analogue scale may be used in which a 10 cm line is drawn and divided into 1 cm portions. At each end of the scale the extremes of the symptoms are noted; for example: no pain—pain unbearable, or unable to eat at all; eating normally, or no vomiting—vomiting continuously. The patient is then asked to mark the point on the scale which corresponds to the severity of his own symptom. Although his method remains subjective it is simple and has been widely used to document the course of the disease.

The general activity of the patient must be assessed, and limiting factors such as pain, breathlessness and weakness need to be carefully documented. It is often useful to know how the patient passes the day: how much is he in bed or in a chair? Can he manage at home and how much help does he need to do so? Can he see to read, work with his hands, write? Such factors can be expressed semiquantitatively by the Karnovsky index (Table 3.1) and the Eastern Co-operative Oncology Group (ECOG) score (Table 3.2); schemes of this kind add nothing to a thorough clinical assessment, but they may be useful in comparing patients when some new therapeutic procedure is being evaluated.

It is important to obtain a full list of drugs being taken, together with their frequency of administration and their effectiveness for the patient. Inadequate relief of symptoms is sometimes due to appropriate drugs inappropriately prescribed. When, towards the end of the interview, some rapport has been

Table 3.1   Karnovsky index of performance status

Normal	100
Minor signs or symptoms	90
Normal activity with effort	80
Unable to carry on normal activity, but cares for self	70
Requires occasional assistance with personal needs	60
Requires considerable assistance and medical care	50
Disabled	40
Severely disabled and hospitalized	30
Very sick: active supportive treatment necessary	20
Moribund	10
Death	0

Table 3.2   ECOG performance status

Grade 0	Fully active, able to carry on all pre-disease performance without restrictions
Grade 1	Restricted in strenuous activity but ambulatory and able to carry out work of a light and sedentary nature, e.g. light housework or office work
Grade 2	Ambulatory and capable of all self-care but unable to carry out any work activity; up and about more than 50% of waking hours
Grade 3	Capable of only limited self-care; confined to bed or chair more than 50% of waking hours
Grade 4	Completely disabled, cannot carry out any self-care, and totally confined to bed or chair

established, the patient should be encouraged to discuss what he himself knows, thinks and fears about his condition (see Chapter 4). Talking to the patient's relatives is essential.

The physical examination

Although this will concentrate on the points raised in the preceding history, it must be sufficiently general to reveal any problem not mentioned by the patient. The following points are particularly important:

1. The entire *skin surface* should be examined to exclude superficial recurrent or metastatic tumour. Pressure sores and breaks in the skin—over the vertebral spines, sacrum, ischial tuberosities, ankles, elbows—must be recorded.

2. Examination of the *mouth, tongue and pharynx* will indicate the state of hydration and the presence of local lesions such as ulceration and fungal infections, notably by Candida.

3. *In the alimentary system.* The examiner should concentrate on gastric distension, incipient bowel obstruction, abdominal masses, ascites, functioning of surgical stomata and hepatomegaly. A rectal examination is essential in all patients to check for faecal impaction and perianal infection.

4. Examination of the lungs, heart, blood pressure and peripheral pulses may clarify the breathlessness and chest pain of which patients often complain.

5. Careful neurological examination may establish the basis for local symptoms such as pain or impending paraplegia. The distinction between widespread intracranial metastatic disease and neuropsychiatric disorders can be extremely difficult.

The history and physical examination of the patient have been discussed here in some detail, but their importance is worth repeating: without an adequate description and at least partial identification of a patient's symptoms and signs, treatment cannot be effectively planned and no valid assessment can be made of therapeutic responses.

Is the diagnosis correct?

The question must now be asked: Are the symptoms and signs elicited attributable to malignant disease, or do they reflect some unrelated disease progress which is occurring coincidentally in a patient with cancer? In such patients, *sinister symptoms are sometimes simple*. An accurate history and physical examination may be sufficient to decide the point, but additional simple investigations are sometimes required. The following patients provide some examples.

1. A 55-year-old male with inoperable gastric carcinoma, diagnosed 6 months previously and treated by chemotherapy. His general practitioner telephoned to say that the patient had developed pulmonary metastases and that he would be cared for at home in what was described as a terminal phase. The patient was, however, admitted to hospital where he was found to have a cough and purulent sputum; a chest x-ray showed changes of chronic bronchitis only. He was treated with antibiotics and was well enough to return home after 5 days. He is alive 1 year later.

2. A 50-year-old male with advanced non-Hodgkin's lymphoma of the stomach which had been successfully treated by chemotherapy. The abdominal mass disappeared, the patient was free of tumour on investigation, and treatment was stopped. The general practitioner telephoned to say that the patient had developed severe backache; he assumed that the patient now had disseminated tumour and would require no further active treatment. The patient was, however, seen at the out-patient clinic. He was still clinically tumour free, and the history and physical signs suggested a prolapsed intervertebral disc. Bone scan and skeletal surveys were negative and the disc lesion was treated conservatively. The patient remains well 18 months later.

3. A 60-year-old female with bilateral breast carcinoma and evidence of secondary spread, presenting with jaundice and right upper abdominal pain. The initial diagnosis was of liver metastases, but further investigations revealed gallstones and the patient had a cholecystectomy. She remained pain-free until her death from disseminated cancer 9 months later.

4. Male, aged 60, with oesophageal carcinoma which had been resected 2 months previously. Patient presented with dysphagia, suggesting locally recurrent tumour. Endoscopy showed a non-absorbable suture in the lumen at the site of the anastomosis. This material was removed, the dysphagia was relieved, and he remains well 1 year later.

These four patients illustrate a number of points. Their symptoms, though not related directly to their malignant disease, were serious and required prompt treatment in their own right. Secondly, relief of these symptoms improved the quality of the patient's life even though the underlying malignant disease continued to advance. Thirdly, they illustrate certain attitudes of doctors to patients with advanced malignancy. There is a sharp contrast between the clinician who says merely that a patient has advanced disease and requires sedation, and the clinician who says that a patient has advanced disease and requires symptom control—and at the same time recognizes the need for the nature of that symptom to be explored in more detail.

Investigative procedures in the terminally ill

This is a debatable topic. Some clinicians argue that such patients should be treated on a purely symptomatic basis. In many instances, access to laboratory or radiological facilities may be difficult or impossible. Within a few days of death, investigative procedures might be regarded as positively unethical.

At some point the clinician must surely ask himself: '*Why* has my patient developed this symptom? And if I understood it more fully, could it not be treated more effectively?' Two points must, however, be clearly stated. Investigative procedures should never be used as grounds for delaying symptomatic treatment; and the investigations chosen should be directed specifically to particular symptoms.

It is obvious that the type of investigation will be determined by the place where the patient is being treated; but some examples of simple, readily available procedures and their applications are given below:

1. *Haemoglobin estimation*. Breathlessness, weakness and fatigue in some severely anaemic patients may be relieved by blood transfusion (see later; also Chapter 6). Such relief will be only transitory but it may be suitable for a particular patient at a particular time in his illness.

2. *Characterization of infections*. Asymptomatic infections require no investigation. Infection causing severe symptoms should usually be treated: isolation of organisms and determination of their antibiotic sensitivities will be done in the usual way. It is improbable that the treatment of serious intercurrent infections materially prolongs life, but the patient will be more comfortable. Major infections occurring as an obvious terminal event should be treated symptomatically (see Chapter 6).

3. *Measurement of serum electrolytes* may be useful in a few instances. Hypercalcaemia, in particular, is worth detecting and correcting (see later; also Chapters 5 and 6).

4. *Radiological investigations* may be considered when appropriate. They should not be carried out routinely.

The value of research in patients with terminal illness

It is only by asking questions, and attempting to solve them, that advances can be made in the practical management of advanced malignant disease. In many instances we still lack basic information on the mechanisms of symptom production and their control (see Chapter 2). It is possible to justify clinical research on these grounds alone, but two questions are paramount: are unnecessary investigations being performed? and are patients suffering needlessly?

Controlled clinical trials

For symptoms such as nausea or anorexia, it is still not clear which mode of therapy is most appropriate; it may be necessary to carry out a study to determine optimal therapy. This topic is discussed further in Chapter 5.

Problem-orientated research

Many specific symptoms such as pain still need to be studied in depth. The form of investigation may involve a patient in procedures which do not contribute directly to his management; it is thus essential that he is fully aware of the purpose of the study and gives his informed consent, and that he receives effective symptomatic therapy at all times.

Investigations involving particular scientific disciplines

The clinician may, for example, have a special interest in biochemical aspects of malignant disease and he may wish to look further into mechanisms of (say) hypercalcaemia or ectopic hormone secretion. The pharmacologist may be interested in drug interactions, an extremely important area when so many patients have multiple drug therapy. Again, such investigations may not directly benefit individual patients; but if carried out in an ethical way they may contribute to a greater understanding of the underlying processes of advanced malignant diseases and their possible palliation.

Has conventional therapy been used to the full?

Surgery; Radiotherapy; Chemotherapy and hormone therapy

These are all discussed elsewhere (see Chapters 7–9) but it is worth noting here that there is an essential difference between the use of conventional methods of anti-cancer therapy in patients with early disease, and in those with terminal disease. In the first circumstance, treatment is used to eradicate tumour in the hope of cure; in the latter it is used for palliation. As modes of treatment become more effective, particularly in the use of combined methods, the point at which there is a change of tactic—from active anticancer therapy to active symptomatic care—becomes less easy to define. It is essential not to regard the 'care' or 'cure' situations in too rigid a manner; the important thing to establish is that the patient is in the appropriate category at each stage of the disease.

Has the time for terminal care been reached?

The fundamental question must be answered for each individual patient on an assessment of some or all of the following factors:

> Symptomatology.
> Evidence for advanced, progressing disease.
> Inability to treat the disease by conventional means, or the failure to respond to therapy.
> Psychological attitude of the patient.

Great difficulties may be encountered in assessing individual cases. A patient may complain of severe, incapacitating pain and yet not have rapidly progressive disease or evidence of clinical deterioration. Conversely, a patient may have advanced, progressive disease, and yet he remains reasonably well, able to work and to function fairly normally. It must be emphasized that advanced metastatic disease is not, in itself, a reliable index of terminal illness. Indeed, some patients, regarded as having far-advanced terminal disease, may remain stable for long periods of time. It is essential that such cases are reviewed regularly, the diagnosis confirmed, and more aggressive antitumour measures reinstituted where appropriate: *continued assessment is the key to appropriate care*. It is also essential at times that the clinician seek a second opinion. This is in no sense a gesture of defeat, but rather an acknowledgement of the difficulty of the problem and the fluidity, in individual cases, of the 'cure'/'care' situations—which can be summarized as cure $\rightleftharpoons$ care (see Chapter 1).

Some systemic changes in patients with terminal cancer

The patient with terminal malignant disease often presents an extremely complex clinical picture. The major symptoms are discussed in Chapter 6; here, we shall stress some of the underlying systemic changes associated with terminal illness which may make management of such symptoms more difficult (see Chapter 2).

Cachexia

This common symptom complex is associated with loss of weight, decreases in body fat, protein and carbohydrate, increased basal metabolic rate and abnormal iron metabolism.

The patient presents clinically with weakness and tiredness associated with weight loss. The aetiology is complex. Cachexia may be consequent upon anorexia, nausea or vomiting, or on gastrointestinal obstruction. It may be compounded by loss of body fluids in association with bleeding or malignant ulcers. Intestinal malabsorption may be involved (see below). The tumour itself may play a part, either by its increased demand for essential nutrients or, more subtly, by synthesizing and releasing products which cause the metabolic changes (see Chapter 2).

Apart from the weakness and tiredness associated with cachexia, there are other serious problems. Such patients are metabolically and nutritionally abnormal, and they may metabolize drugs in a different way from normal individuals; drug efficacy may therefore be modified (see later).

Malabsorption

Malabsorption has frequently been described in patients with cancer, either as a primary event or as a consequence of previous treatment. Repeated courses of chemotherapy or radiotherapy to the abdomen may, for example, induce villous atrophy. Previous surgical treatment of intra-abdominal neoplasms may have been performed with bypass or resection of segments of small bowel.

Malabsorption has serious consequences for the patient. He may develop impaired absorption of essential nutrients, including vitamins. Vitamin deficiency may be associated with skin and mucosal lesions and also anaemia; correction of such deficiencies will be symptomatically beneficial. Several of the vitamins are involved in drug metabolism, and vitamin deficiencies will modify drug efficacy. In addition, absorption of drugs may be delayed or actually impaired. When patients do not respond as expected to drug therapy—for example, in pain control—attention should be given to malabsorption, and the drug given parenterally for a trial period.

Influence of previous treatment

Previous surgery of the tumour may result in residual anatomical or functional impairment to adjacent normal tissues. Such damage may be unimportant when a patient is tolerably well; but it becomes more significant when he is terminally ill. Radiotherapy and cytotoxic drugs may also induce tissue damage which declares itself at a later stage. Cystitis following radiotherapy or treatment with cyclophosphamide is difficult to control; so, too, is the proctitis that may follow pelvic irradiation. Drug therapy may be associated with severe bone marrow toxicity and immune depression, thus favouring infections (see later). Many side effects may be encountered in patients treated with high doses of corticosteroids, particularly weakness, glycosuria, osteoporosis and peptic ulceration.

Renal problems in advanced cancer

These are associated with direct involvement of the kidneys or lower urinary tract by tumour or, in a small percentage of cases, with deposition of immune complexes in the glomerular basement membrane. There is deterioration of renal function with rising blood urea and serum creatinine levels. Drug excretion in such patients may be delayed and consideration should always be given to this possibility when severe and unexplained side-effects of drugs occur. 'Pre-renal' uraemia, due to failing renal perfusion, is a frequent late terminal finding.

Hepatic involvement in advanced cancer

Liver metastases, often massive, are common in many patients with advanced cancer. In addition to causing the specific symptoms and signs of jaundice, itch, nausea and sometimes profound anorexia, more general consequences may ensue. Protein synthesis is decreased with widespread liver involvement. There is a fall in serum albumin levels, which may be associated with peripheral oedema. Drug metabolism may be altered. The synthesis of components of the blood coagulation system, including fibrinogen, may be affected. Rapid hepatic enlargement or bleeding within liver metastases is often associated with severe local pain.

Haematological problems in the terminally ill

Patients with advanced malignant disease are frequently anaemic. Mild asymptomatic anaemias require no investigation or treatment. Severe anaemia may require therapy. The cause is usually obvious; for example, bleeding from a tumour or marrow invasion and little investigation is needed. Blood transfusion is likely to improve symptoms for only a short time before the anaemia recurs. This short time can, however, mean the difference between a patient being treated at home or being treated in hospital, and there are individual occasions when even one week-end at home, made possible by blood trans-fusion, is justified for some domestic or social occasion.

Coagulation abnormalities, involving either bleeding or disseminated intra-vascular coagulation, may be encountered in terminal illness. They do not require active management. Intramuscular injections should be avoided in these circumstances in case they cause painful bleeding.

Other biochemical changes

Hypercalcaemia occurs more frequently in advanced malignant disease than is often supposed. Its symptoms include confusion, abdominal pain, restlessness and irritability, progressing to drowsiness and coma. Adequate hydration will control this symptom complex in about half the cases. Where this is not success-ful, prednisolone or cortisol may be used together with oral phosphate. In the small number of patients who do not respond to these methods, intravenous mithramycin may be successful. Hypercalcaemia can simulate intracranial metastases and, as it is a treatable condition, it should not be overlooked.

Hyperuricaemia may occur, caused by anticancer therapy. As it can result in painful gouty tophi, it may merit active management. Phenylbutazone is given in the acute situation, and allopurinol as a preventive measure.

Electrolyte imbalance is common in patients with repeated vomiting or exces-sive fluid loss, and such patients are often severely dehydrated. Where it occurs shortly before death, intravenous fluid replacement is inappropriate. But it may be necessary to consider such measures in patients in whom the acute problem can be resolved—for example, by palliative surgery (see Chapter 9).

Peripheral oedema in the cancer patient has a complex aetiology. It may be related to low serum albumin levels, electrolyte abnormalities, tumour involve-ment of lymph nodes and lymphatic obstruction, renal failure or myocardial failure. Oedema of this type is often resistant to therapy; treatment with diuretics or cardiac glycosides may bring undesirable side-effects, and the possibilities of deleterious drug interactions should not be forgotten.

Ectopic hormone secretion may be encountered with several tumours, especially some carcinomas of the lung. Ectopic ACTH secretion is associated with the symptoms and signs of Cushing's syndrome. Excessive secretion of antidiuretic hormone (ADH) results in electrolyte abnormalities associated with water intoxication: serum sodium levels fall and the patient becomes weak, confused and inco-ordinated. Coma and convulsions may occur. The condition can be corrected by fluid restriction and occasionally by the use of hypertonic solutions. More recently Lithium or demeclocycline have been used successfully. Excess parathyroid hormone secretion may result in hyper-calcaemia (see above).

The importance of these somewhat esoteric biochemical problems does not, in the present context, lie in the elucidation of the underlying abnormality; rather, it lies in the exploitation of this knowledge to improve the quality of care given to patients with advanced malignant disease. Confusion, rest-lessness, nausea and vomiting may all result from these biochemical abnor-malities; if they are corrected, the patient will feel better and the quality of his re-maining life will be improved. By the simple expedient of measuring the serum electrolytes, calcium and uric acid, any abnormalities noted can often be treated.

Confusion in the patient with terminal cancer

The patient with advanced cancer may be confused and restless in the end stages of disease as a result of several factors:

Intracerebral metastases. These are a common cause of confusion, usually associated with neurological signs and an abnormal EEG or brain scan. Temporary benefit may result from the use of dexamethasone (see Chapters 5 and 6).

Drug overdosage. It is essential to review the drug history of the confused patient. He may be suffering from excess sedation or the inappropriate use of tranquillizers.

Biochemical disturbances. Some of these have already been discussed. It is worth considering whether the confused, restless patient has an acute vitamin deficiency, particularly of the B group. Wernicke's encephalopathy, which may be confused with cerebral metastases, responds well to intravenous vitamin therapy.

Infection and the immune response

It is now well established that patients with advanced cancer often have depressed immunological responses involving cell-mediated immunity, antibody production or both. Such patients are more prone to infection, sometimes by unusual micro-organisms or organisms which are usually of only minimal pathogenicity.

Drug metabolism and drug interactions

Throughout this chapter reference has been made to anomalies of drug metabolism consequent upon malabsorption, metabolic abnormalities, or renal and liver failure.

Drugs used in the patient with terminal illness include a wide variety of analgesics, antiemetics and sedatives. The use of such drugs, in combination, may result in significant interactions. Metoclopramide, for example, delays gastric emptying and may delay the effect of other drugs. Monoamine oxidase inhibitors interact with pethidine and the tricylic antidepressants, and they should be used together only with the greatest care. Aspirin may interact with probenecid and methotrexate. Many of the drug combinations used in clinical practice have unknown interactions and the clinician must always be on the watch for adverse results.

Physical aspects of terminal care in children

The plan of management outlined in this chapter applies equally well to children as to adults. The metabolic problems which occur in children are often more acute, but their remarkable resilience makes them able to withstand these more readily. Inevitably, the decision that a child has reached a terminal state is made more reluctantly. There is a tendency to 'treat till the last' in the hope that something will work; consequently the time during which symptomatic care only is given may be relatively short.

Nevertheless, whatever the patient's age, the over-riding requirement is attention to detail—to the causes behind the symptoms and, above all, to a continual assessment which ceases only with the patient's death.

References and further reading

BROWNE, Sir Thomas. (1672) *Religio medici* pti, p. 39.
FRY, Christopher (1954). *The Dark is Light Enough*. Oxford University Press; London.

Cachexia and Nutritional Problems

COSTA, G. (1963). Cachexia, the metabolic component of neoplastic diseases. *Progress in Experimental Tumour Research* 3, 321.
THEOGLIDES, A. (1972). Pathogenesis of cachexia in cancer. *Cancer* 29, 484.
DeWYS, W. (1970). Working conference on anorexia and cachexia of neoplastic disease. *Cancer Research* 30, 2816.

Ectopic Hormones

ROSS, E. J. (1972). Endocrine and metabolic manifestations of cancer. *British Medical Journal* 1, 735.
RATCLIFFE, J. G. and REES, L. H. (1974). Clinical manifestations of ectopic hormone production. *British Journal of Hospital Medicine* II, 685.

Hypercalcaemia

COOMBES, R. C., WARD, M. K., GREENBERG, P. B., HILLYARD, C. J., TULLICH, B. R., MORRISION, R. and JOPLIN, G. F. (1976). Calcium metabolism in cancer. *Cancer* 38, 2111.
Symposium (1977). Hypercalcaemia in malignant disease. *Proceedings of the Royal Society of Medicine* 70, 191.

Haematological Problems

ANNER, R. M. and DREWINKO, B. (1977). Frequency and significance of bone marrow involvement by metastatic solid tumours. *Cancer* 39, 1337.
PECK, S. D. and REIQUAM, C. W. (1977). Disseminated intravascular coagulation in cancer patients: supportive evidence. *Cancer* 39, 1337.

Drug-related Problems

ALVARES, A. P., ANDERSON, K. E., CONNEY, A. H. and KAPPAS, A. (1976). Interactions between nutritional factors and drug biotransformations in man. *Proceedings of the National Academy of Sciences of the USA* 73, 2501.
RUMACH, B. H., HOLTZMAN, J. and CHASE, H. P. (1973). Hepatic drug metabolism and protein malnutrition. *Journal of Pharmacology and Experimental Therapeutics* 186, 441.
ZANNONI, V. G. and RIKANS, L. E. (1976). Ascorbic acid and drug detoxification. *Trends in Biochemical Sciences* 1, 126.

Immunological Problems

CURRIE, G. A. (1974). *Cancer and the Immune Response*. Edward Arnold; London.

4

Psychological Aspects

C. Murray Parkes

Editorial note

Hinton's paper 'Talking with people about to die' summarizes the comments of 60 patients receiving care for terminal cancer made to him about their discussions with doctors and nurses. Of these, 40 had some awareness of dying and none disapproved of open discussion. Of the 21 reporting little or no truthful conversation with the staff, 9 were critical but the other 12 were not dissatisfied, including some aware of their prognosis (Hinton, 1974). His 1963 paper included assessments of the insight of 102 dying patients, when he found that 50 per cent had a shrewd idea of the seriousness of their illness when he first met them and that 75 per cent indicated they knew that they were dying as the time drew near.

Witzel reported interviews with 110 patients shortly before their death and found them resigned, with little or no fear, though expressing no desire for details about their illness. He compared them with a control group with serious but not fatal illness. The second group wanted information about their condition and feared death, though few thought they would actually die (Witzel, 1975).

McIntosh has recently reported on a year's study in a cancer ward where 'the cornerstone of the doctors' philosophy on telling was the belief that the great majority of the patients "should not be told".' He found that the overwhelming majority of the patients knew or suspected they had a malignancy, but that 70 per cent of them did not want any confirmation of their prognosis. He did not consider that these patients anticipated that they would adjust better to their illness if they were told (McIntosh, 1977).

Graeme writes of 'the broad road of daily encouragement and support' which lies between 'stark realities on the one hand and the silent evasion or hearty *bonhomie* on the other' (Graeme, 1975), and finds many patients do not want confirmation until the end is near.

The appeal for quantitative studies to add to the 'anecdotal approach' has given us valuable information but not the clear guidelines which some may have hoped for. We still have to attempt to meet with each individual patient as one person with another and try to assess what his needs may be at that particular moment. These needs may change throughout the progress of the illness. One week-end, as duty doctor, I attempted with the help of the nursing staff to assess the insight and acceptance of all our 50 in-patients. At the same time, two members of our Domiciliary team made a similar assessment of 20 patients who had been visited during the last 3 days. We both found a situation much more akin to Hinton's findings than McIntosh's; but it was not a static situation. For example, in one ward among 11 patients I talked with I found 7 patients with clear insight into their condition, living day by day with life as it came and relating easily and appropriately with their families and the staff. There were 4 patients who seemed to be denying the fact of their obviously deteriorating condition (something it is perfectly possible to do in St Christopher's Hospice). Discussing these same 4 patients with the ward doctor a week later, I discovered that 2 of them had died, having quietly faced the approach of death with acceptance. The Domiciliary team, whose patients were on the whole at an earlier stage of their illness had also observed several similar changes in the 7 days since their first assessment.

We are involved with people whose situation, insight and needs change constantly. Parkes describes these changes with experience and understanding and, unlike many of the writers in this field, includes the family in his perspective. This has been discussed already (Chapter 1), for our concern must include the way the family as a group comes to terms with this situation and faces the future.

The comment of the husband of one of our long-stay patients, who has spent 8 years visiting in our wards and is no mean observer in his own right, sums up the experience of St Christopher's Hospice. 'By the end of about a week, when they know they won't have any more pain, most of them begin to live quite happily and face what is coming as it comes. But there are a few who never want to look at it and they don't have to.'

'No more pain'. The competent control of symptoms is essential. The journey into understanding and acceptance which Dr Parkes describes would be grievously hampered by unrelieved physical problems.

'The human claim to a portion of divinity rests safely on the capacity of men to suffer, on the genius by which they transcend their suffering.' (Hutchinson, 1952.) We cannot take away the suffering of weakness and parting, but we can do much to help our patients to transcend it if we lift many of its physical elements from them. Here we see courage, patience and endurance, and finally, as Worcester noted, that 'Death is almost always preceded by a perfect willingness to die.' (Worcester, 1935.)

Parkes shows us that the family, too, can be helped towards a willingness to live on afterwards.

References

GRAEME, P. (1975). Support for the dying patient and the family. In: Symposium on *Cancer, the Patient and the Family*. Ed. by R. W. Raven. Sherratt; Altrincham.
HINTON, J. (1963). Mental and physical distress in the dying. *Quarterly Journal of Medicine* 1.
HINTON, J. (1974). Talking with people about to die. *British Medical Journal* 2, 25.
HUTCHINSON, R. C. (1952). *Recollections of a Journey*. Cassell; London.
McINTOSH, J. (1977). *Communication and Awareness in a Cancer Ward*. Croom Helm; London. Prodist; New York.
WITZEL, L. (1975). Behaviour of the dying patient. *British Medical Journal* 2, 81.
WORCESTER, A. (1935). *The Care of the Aged, the Dying and the Dead*. Thomas; Springfield, Illinois. (1961). Blackwells, Oxford. Reprinted 1977, under *The Literature of Death and Dying*, Arno Press, New York.

'How little the real sufferings of illness are known and understood. How little does anyone in good health fancy him or even *herself* into the life of a sick person.'
    (Nightingale, 1946)

Time to live

A knowledge of the psychosocial aspects of dying is as important to those who care for people approaching death as is a knowledge of anatomy to the surgeon. In a sense, a cancer can extend beyond the person who harbours it, and any approach to understanding must embrace the entire social unit.

One could say the same of any other potentially fatal illness, but cancer has one great advantage over most of the rest—it gives us time. In one study of people who died from cancer in two London boroughs, 18 per cent were still under investigation or active treatment at the time of death. The rest were known by their relatives to have come to the end of active curative treatment *before* they died (Parkes, 1978). They had received a period of care, much of it at home, during which the patient, the family and care-givers had an opportunity to come to terms with the realities of the illness and to prepare themselves for the changes in the family which would come about when the patient died. In this chapter we shall examine how it is possible to do this and how doctors, nurses and others can help.

Both clinical experience and systematic studies confirm the importance of time in enabling people to prepare for disasters. The Harvard Bereavement Study showed that the death of a husband or wife under the age of 45 had a much more devastating effect if the death was sudden and unexpected than if it had been gradual and anticipated. The diagnosis of malignant disease, as opposed to other causes of death, was significantly correlated with better adjustment to bereavement in the spouse a year later (Glick, Weiss and Parkes, 1974; Parkes, 1976).

Time is of little use if it is not properly employed. For the family and for the patient the period of terminal care can be a time of growth and shared preparation, or it can be a time of defeat and mutual destruction. Used well, it can see the fulfilment and completion of a marriage. Used badly, it can mar the memory of good relationships and undermine the health of the survivors for years to come.

It is clearly imperative for us, the care-givers, to try to help patient and family to make the best use of the time that remains to them. This is the main aim of terminal care and the most important single service which we have to offer. If we fail to recognize the opportunity which terminal care represents in terms of family growth and development we have nothing to offer but palliation, the mitigation of suffering by symptom relief alone. This type of palliative care is purely negative.

The starting point of any positive approach to terminal care must lie in the care-givers' ability to understand the nature of the problems confronting the family. The family (which includes the patient) *is* the unit of care, and the fact that it may be the patient who has sought our help gives us no excuse for ignoring the rest of the social unit which has been invaded by cancer. I would suggest that the traditional injunction to young doctors to 'treat the whole patient' be expanded to 'treat the whole family'. This implies that we must meet the family, or at least those members who are most closely involved, and attempt to open an effective channel of communication with them.

Traditional psychiatric diagnosis is of little value in this field. It will be of no help to a dying man to label him as suffering from 'a depression', nor will his wife benefit from being told that she is suffering from 'an anxiety state'. Similarly, in deciding how to help a dying man, it is more appropriate to attempt to understand the problems to which his illness has given rise and to work out a way of helping him with these problems than to prescribe a 'treatment' as if the problems were themselves an illness.

Occasionally, malignant disease, or its medical or surgical consequences, may damage the brain and there is then a need to differentiate the symptoms of organic mental disorder from the emotional accompaniments of the disease. However, the symptoms of the organic disorder produced by malignant disease are no different from those of organic disorder arising from other causes; both are described in textbooks of neurology and psychiatry.

In considering the psychological aspects of malignant disease a different frame of reference is required, and I have preferred to adopt the viewpoint which has emerged from studies of bereavement and other major life changes in recent years. This identifies two main components as regular occurrences whenever a person is faced with the need to abandon one set of assumptions about the world and to develop another. On the one hand there is fear, apprehension and attempts to ward off the dangers which may yet be averted; on the other hand there is grief, mourning and a tendency to move towards the realization of the new situation which is emerging.

In the face of advancing malignant disease, these two components are seen in family members as well as patients, and they influence all the interactions between care-givers and cared-for. For convenience we shall consider first how they affect the patient, and then move on to consider the other members of the patient's family before looking at some of the implications for the organization of the care-giving team.

Fear and the patient

Effective communication about matters of life and death is often hedged round with difficulties, most of them caused by the fear which such communication evokes in the patient, the family and the care-givers themselves. Our starting point for the understanding of this situation must therefore be to examine the fear.

Fear is a natural reaction to danger and it is easy to understand why it occurs when a family member is threatened with death. We are familiar with the neurophysiological accompaniments of fear and can appreciate their biological function in the fight/flight responses classically described by Cannon (1929). What is less generally recognized is the extent to which the expression of fear often becomes blocked, distorted or fragmented in a patient faced with the prospect of incurable disease.

This distortion of fear was illustrated clearly by a woman in her middle 50s. She was proud of the fact that she had forced her doctor to tell her that she had cancer, and that she had no fear of dying. Her only complaint at the time of her admission to St Christopher's Hospice was concerned with her eyes. Every time she looked in the mirror she was upset by the expression on her face. This expression contrasted with her protested lack of fear, for her upper eyelids were retracted and she gave the appearance of being terrified. The ward staff tried to reassure her and give her the support which she needed but within 24 hours she ran away by discharging herself home. During the ensuing weeks her medical attendants and her family found it hard to support her and cope with the continued deterioration in her physical condition. However, patience and concerned care paid off and before long she was accepting help from the Home Care nurses from the Hospice. As her physical status became worse, her mental status improved and eventually she asked to return to the Hospice. On readmission her frightened stare had passed and she was relaxed and seemed delighted to be back. The ward staff were astonished at the change in her demeanour which remained friendly and serene until she died peacefully a few weeks later.

This case illustrates clearly the way in which fear can be intellectually denied but remain physiologically active. It also illustrates the interesting paradox that as the danger becomes greater the fear may grow less. This progression can never be taken for granted but, if circumstances of care are good, it occurs with sufficient frequency to encourage the nurses and doctors to do all in their power to further it.

In this example it was the existence of fear which was denied. In other cases fear is accepted but its cause is denied or displaced. Thus a person may admit to feeling generally anxious but he is unable to recognize any cause for his anxiety. Alternatively, the fear may be focused on a particular symptom or circumstance which has little to do with its real cause. Some people can feel fear on behalf of somebody else, a husband or wife whose life is affected by their illness, but deny any fear on their own behalf. Others attempt to control their fear by avoiding any thought or utterance which will evoke it; they restrict communication to trivialities and pointedly ignore any opportunity which doctors or others may give them to talk about their illness.

These defence mechanisms are not confined to the patients. Family members and even doctors and nurses regularly avoid or deny recognition of the danger which the patient is in as if, by so doing, they could thereby avoid the danger itself. Such avoidance of reality is usually justified on the grounds that there is no point in upsetting people. 'Recognizing the danger will not make it go away. Why not pretend that it isn't there?'

This may lead to a conspiracy between the family and the medical attendants to deceive the patient into thinking that he is getting better—a benevolent conspiracy often upset by the disease process itself. Faced with increasing evidence of his physical deterioration the patient may eventually conclude that, if everybody is trying to deny the facts, then the facts must be truly terrible. This only increases his fear. As one patient sardonically remarked, 'I'm relieved to hear that I'm not dying of anything serious'!

Responding to the patient's fear and anxiety

When a person has an illness likely to prove fatal, it is too easy for us to imagine that we understand his anxiety and to discourage further communication about this distressing topic. He may say, 'I am frightened of dying,' and we hastily murmur, 'Yes, of course,' and change to some more cheerful subject. Yet the dying patient can fear many things and a more appropriate response may be, 'Are you? Well tell me just what you mean by that.' Encouraged to talk further the patient will then express fears, some of which may be quite needless. Many people imagine death to be an agonizing disintegration—they may need to be reassured that the moment of death from cancer is almost invariably peaceful.

Others see death as the ultimate loss of control and need assurance that they will not be a burden. Some are frightened of what will become of others after their death and at a certain point (though not too early) they may need to be assured that wife, children and other dependents can cope on their own. But in all cases the essential requirement is to show interest and to listen to what the patient has to say. The slightest drawing back on our part will be recognized by the patient as a confirmation of his fears and a sign that he can expect no help from us.

The commonest fear expressed by patients with terminal cancer is fear of separation from people, home, job and the like (Parkes, 1973). This is a reasonable fear and a proper cause for grief. To some extent the grief can be mitigated if it is shared with us and with others. Separation anxiety will also be reduced if members of the family are encouraged to stay close to the patient and no restrictions are placed upon them visiting him in hospital. Likewise, every opportunity should be given to patients in hospital to visit their homes if only for a few hours at a time. But in the end the grief of separation must be borne.

Less common are fears of failing to complete some life task or fulfil some obligation. People who have spent years working to achieve some end which will never be accomplished, or couples who have been staying together in the hope that a difficult relationship would one day improve, find it hard to accept the fact that their hopes will not be realized. In such instances, as in many others, anger is an understandable reaction and the patient may need to rage against God and man before he can take stock of the value of the life which remains to him. Any attempt on our part to combat the patient's rage by rational argument or reassurance is likely to fail and may be taken as a rejection. It is better to 'bow before the storm' and wait until the patient is ready to take a more positive view.

Linked with this is the fear of death as a punishment. It seems to me that the concept of death as something done to a person which can be viewed as fair or unfair according to his desserts is the modern equivalent of the fear of judgment which played so large a part at the deathbeds of earlier times. This is sometimes expressed as a fear of the unknown. But if we have faith in the known we have less need to fear the unknown. Not many people today express a fear of hell or a hope of heaven, but there are still many who find it easier to approach death because of some belief in an ultimate purpose which they may or may not call God.

These examples hardly do justice to the complexity of the problems which are encountered in our day-to-day work with people who are near to the ending of their lives; but we do not need to feel pessimistic. If the fear is unrealistic we must provide reassurance; if it is realistic we must be prepared to help the patient to confront the losses which are impending and to express the grief which is appropriate to each loss. By demonstrating our willingness to share the patient's grief we help him to accept it himself. Thus we gently help the patient to move from a position of avoidance towards a position of acceptance.

Grief and the patient

The strongest argument against benevolent conspiracies is not that they do not work (they sometimes do) but that they are rarely necessary. Experience has repeatedly shown that if a person is given the opportunity to learn the facts of his case, little by little, at his own pace, and provided he is encouraged to share with others the feelings which these facts evoke, and provided that others are not constantly feeding back to him their own fears, he will move progressively closer to a full realization of the situation without suffering overwhelming panic or despair.

The process of realization

This realization follows much the same pattern as the process of realization (grief) which follows any major loss (Parkes, 1972a). Grief arises in any situation in which a person is forced by circumstances to give up one view of the world and accept another for which he is not prepared. The griever moves progressively from a state of incomprehension or numbness ('I can't believe it's true'), to a period of intense inner struggle in which awareness of the reality of death conflicts with a strong impulse to recover the lost person or world in some form or other. This is followed by a phase of dejection and hopelessness in which the grieving person is aware of the discrepancy between his inner model of the world and the world which now exists. Finally, little by little, a new set of assumptions is built up to replace those that are now redundant. The widow begins to think of herself as a widow, the man who has a disabling illness stops thinking of himself as a provider. In a sense both of them have to discover a new identity.

The transition is by no means smooth, and people tend to oscillate across these phases of grief. For a long time anything which brings the person or world which has been lost strongly to mind has the power to evoke another pang of grief, an episode of acute pining in which the urge to recover the lost person or world returns yet again. Hence people will say, 'It doesn't end.' On the other hand, the frequency and intensity of the pangs of grief grow gradually less. Most people who have suffered a major loss eventually experience a regaining of strength which encourages them to use words such as 'recovery' as if they had been through some kind of sickness; other terms which are equally appropriate are 'reintegration' or 'acceptance'.

The dying patient's grief

For the patient who is approaching the end of his life the sickness of grief can complicate the physical sickness from which he is suffering; we have all heard of people who, on learning that their situation was 'hopeless', turned their face to the wall and died after a rapid decline. It would seem from anecdotes of this kind that psychological factors can play a part in determining the length of survival. Confirmation of this fact comes from an important study by Weisman and Worden (1975). These investigators calculated the average survival time of patients with various types of incurable cancer. They then compared a group of patients who survived longer than average with another group who died in a shorter period.

'Longevity . . . was significantly correlated with patients who maintain active and mutually responsive relationships, provided that the intensity of demands was not so extreme as to alienate people responsible for the patients' care.' On the other hand, 'Shorter survival was found among cancer patients who reflected long-standing alienation, deprivation, depression and destructive relationships, which extended into the terminal stage of life. These attitudes of patients were expressed in despondency, desire to die, contemplation of suicide, inordinate complaints, all of which heaped more self-defeat and isolation upon themselves.'

Clearly, the interaction between staff and patients is likely to play a major part in survival. It is my own impression that neither denial of the true facts nor rapid confrontation with overwhelming loss is conducive to long survival. More important, the quality of the life of the patient will be better if he has the opportunity to come to terms with his illness a little at a time. The question is not 'Should the doctor tell?' but 'How much is this patient ready to be told at this point in this illness?' We want to avoid the situation in which a person who is unprepared for bad news is told that he must lose everything he values. This situation is more likely to arise if doctors mislead their patients than if they admit from the start that the illness may be serious (see Chapter 1).

In the usual, and most desirable, course of events, the cancer patient is not faced with one massive loss but with a series of disappointments each of which, with proper guidance, he can master before he is confronted with the next. He may need, at first, to realize that his symptoms are going to cause some major disruption in his life. After his first surgical operation he may be faced with lasting disability. If the disease recurs he will probably come to recognize that he is unlikely to return to work and eventually that his long-term plans will need revision. As the illness progresses, it may become appropriate for him to face the fact that he is unlikely to live for as long as he had hoped. If he can do this it will then become easier for him to accept a shorter and shorter prognosis. When, at last, the final stage of the illness is reached, increasing disability seems to reduce the appetite not only for food but for life itself. The last episodes may well be more peaceful and less distressing than any previous phase.

Elizabeth Kübler Ross, in her classical study of the emotional reactions to dying, describes five stages which correspond fairly closely to the phases of realization which are found after bereavement (Ross, 1970). Other writers have criticized this classification on the grounds that many patients do not seem to follow the stages as described (Schulz and Aderman, 1974).

In fairness to Ross, she never claimed that all of her stages must be passed through by every patient; but the fact that she terms them 'stages' leads us to expect a sequence. Ross's stages are: (1) denial and isolation; (2) anger; (3) bargaining; (4) depression; and (5) acceptance. They describe a process of realization with the later stages reflecting a greater recognition of the facts of death. I suspect, however, that one of the reasons why this progression is seldom seen clearly among cancer patients is the irregular and unpredictable character of the disease itself. There is seldom one particular moment when doctors and patient become aware that the patient has a certain limited time to live; even when we think we can guess how long our patients are likely to survive we are usually wrong—to judge from a study of predictions of survival at St Christopher's Hospice (Parkes, 1972b). More often, the patient is faced with a number of disappointments each of which must be grieved before the person is ready to move on to the next. Weisman and Worden (1977, personal communication) call these 'crisis points' and are currently mapping out the 'crisis points' which characterize each major type of cancer. Some of these disappointments may be overcome quite easily while others may severely tax the patient's resources of courage and hope.

A relaxed and contented patient is a great source of reassurance to the family, particularly if he is being nursed at home. Conversely, the patient who is suffering unrelieved distress may place an intolerable burden on the family who may be quite unable to cope with his rage and despair. I have known relationships to break down because of the irritability and anger evoked by severe physical distress.

Fear and the family

The period of terminal care is a most important time for the family. It enables them to prepare for the patient's death and to make restitution to him for the fact of their own survival and for any failures or ambivalence which has previously impaired the relationship. The term 'anticipatory grieving' has been used to describe this process but I think that this is usually a misnomer. A wife whose husband is about to die may experience a great deal of fear and anticipatory anxiety, but her grief will seldom proceed to the point of detachment and she will not make serious plans for her future life. The reasons are twofold. One is that the presence of a sick person strengthens attachment; we all tend to come closer to the helpless and weak. The other is that a plan is psychologically so close to a wish that any plan for life after the patient's death can become a wish. The person who has wished another one dead eventually feels that it was the wish which caused the death, and he may even come to see himself as a murderer.

A dying patient may want to make plans for his nearest relatives and this may be something which they will respect. The dying know, of course, that their wishes are likely to be respected and this gives them a power which may be abused. More appropriately, a person who is close to death will attempt to influence those whom he expects to survive him, not by prescribing what they should or should not do, but by releasing them from any sense of continued obligation to him.

Both patients and family members have their own fears and griefs to face and they may choose to avoid communication with each other about them. Even then, however, each continues to influence the other and any attempt to understand the situation must take this into account. A wife, for instance, may deliberately avoid discussing her husband's illness with a doctor for fear that she will be unable to conceal from her husband any distress to which this communication gives rise. She may, therefore, fail to understand the nature or seriousness of his condition and be unprepared for its outcome. Similarly, a patient may imagine that he is protecting his spouse by concealing from her his awareness of the true state of affairs. The spouse, on the other hand, may be under considerable strain because she is attempting to conceal the same facts from him. In this way both parties are deprived of the chance to share their feelings and to create something positive out of the last chapter of their marriage.

More often than not, patient and family are 'out of step' because the patient is given a more optimistic view of his prospects than are his family. One might expect this to make the family members more distressed than the patient since they have a fuller knowledge of the danger, but in fact family members regularly adopt the psychological defence of postponement as a means of coping with the situation. In order to fulfil their obligations to the patient and provide him with proper care they repress their own grief, adopt a rigorous policy of self-control and behave as if their understanding of illness was the same as the patient's. This inhibition of realization is bought at a price, and many family members are aware of a strong sense of rising inner tension which may be expressed as a fear that they will 'break down'. They may show many of the physiological accompaniments of severe anxiety—eating little, losing weight and sleeping poorly—and it is sometimes necessary to take the patient into hospital simply to give his nearest relatives a rest. A minor tranquillizer such as diazepam by day or nitrazepam at night will often enable a spouse to continue his or her care for the patient, but doctors should be wary of using more powerful drugs which can reduce the ability of the family members to continue their caring functions.

The sad fact is that much of this defensiveness is unnecessary. If only the patient and the family can be helped to share the truth instead of avoiding it, the general level of tension will often be reduced and the need for drugs to reduce emotional tension artificially will diminish. Unfortunately, doctors and nurses usually find it easier to administer the drugs than to take the time to talk with patients and family members in the hope of resolving rather than repressing their problems.

During the terminal stage the primary focus of care is inevitably the patient rather than the family, and family members should not be discouraged from the self-sacrifice which may be their last gift to him. It is easy for doctors and nurses to reassure them that their help is not needed. 'Don't you worry, leave everything to us.' But in doing so we may simply confirm a relative in the belief that he or she is unable to care for the dying person at this most critical time in his life. The wife, who after nursing her husband at home finally realizes that she cannot cope, will feel doubly guilty if the ward staff make her feel an intruder at his bedside and restrict the time which she can spend with him in hospital.

Relatives and patients are usually grateful for the efficient way in which hospital staff take over responsibility for a situation which has become increasingly frightening, but we should not let their gratitude blind us to the importance which each of them will continue to play in the life of the other. At this time it is we, not they, who are the intruders and we should make our intervention as gentle as possible. In a terminal care ward the patient's family are not intruders, nor are they honoured guests; they are an intimate part of the network of care. They are both care-givers and cared-for. They belong in the hospital as of right and their needs must be of paramount importance to us.

The patient's troubles are likely soon to be over but the family's may be just beginning.

Even though family members may be one step ahead of the patient in their awareness of his situation, it does not follow that communication between them is impossible. If we keep them informed of the nature of any information which passes between us and the patient or—better still—involve them in the process of communication so that they help the patient with each step of the way, then the gap between them will be reduced.

Counselling the family

There are few forms of therapy more exacting than counselling a family which includes a dying patient. But it is inspiring to see how family members can grow together at such times. The method of counselling is too personal for a general description to be appropriate but there are a few simple rules which apply whether it is a patient or any close family member who needs our help. Non-verbal communication is as important as verbal—the touch of a hand or a smile at the right moment which implies 'It's all right, you don't need to feel afraid', or the sensitive awareness that this is the moment to remain silent and wait for the truth to sink in and for the next question to emerge.

Confidence in our own ability to cope with the situation in our own way, and confidence in the other person's possibilities, will increase with experience. Awareness of the right moment to lower tension by smiling or encouraging someone to 'cheer up' and the right moment to remain serious when the other is offering you an escape ('You didn't come here to listen to my moaning') will grow if we observe carefully the outcome of our attempts to help. The one essential component is a philosophical or a religious attitude in the counsellor which enables him or her to indicate that although the final phase of life may be 'awful' in the old meaning of the word (filled with awe) it need not be approached with pessimism. If we can see the life which precedes death as a positive time with a meaning to be discovered, then patients and their families will find it easier to do the same. We must, however, allow them to discover their own meanings—we cannot impose our own, however valid they may seem to us. People of a religious faith are in a minority today and for most of us the search for meaning is not expressed in 'religious' language. Even so one can justifiably regard the search as a 'religious' activity since it is concerned with the attempt to relate the significance of an individual life to that of some wider reality.

'Involvement' and 'distancing'

Although I have described the counselling of the family at times of death as exacting, I do not think it is too difficult to be attempted by the majority of people who have chosen to join the care-giving professions. There are, however, certain peculiarities about the circumstances in which death now takes place and certain aspects of the training of doctors and nurses which militate against this. It is almost as if the health care system, by dedicating itself to the saving of life, had ruled death out of order. Or, as Eric Cassell put it in a recent paper, 'Death is now a failure of technology' (1974). The doctor's basic medical training teaches him to see the human body as a series of mechanisms which are liable to disorder. The case demonstration method of teaching at the bedside educates the young doctor to see his fellow human beings as 'the cancer in the end bed' and teaches him how to communicate with his colleagues *about* the patient without communicating *with* the patient at all. The dying patient is commonly omitted from discussion altogether.

Nurses learn that it is not permitted for them to discuss serious issues with a patient, and they are encouraged to model themselves on the brisk, efficient, senior who sees it as a virtue not to get 'emotionally involved'. Unlike trainee nurses, medical students seldom see 'emotional involvement' as a problem, probably because they rarely get to know a patient well enough for it to become a risk. However, for the nurse or social worker whose work brings her closer to her patients for longer periods of time, there is always the 'danger' of a relationship developing.

I do not think we can avoid this issue. Human relationships are dangerous. When we get attached to our patients we begin to suffer with them and we may even become involved to the point where we are overwhelmed by our own distress and become useless to them. Although this is true I do not think it justifies the extreme distancing which is encouraged in many teaching hospitals.

In all social situations the question of 'appropriate distance' arises. We are constantly monitoring the physical and mental distance which governs effective and useful communication. Some people are bad at distancing—either they stand too close and assume an intimacy which does not exist, or they put up barriers and repel attempts to 'make contact'.

In general the person who is feeling frightened or insecure has a greater need of close physical contact with people he can trust than the person who is strong and independent. If we are to support a family through the hard times of terminal illness, it will usually be necessary for us to achieve a closeness which is unusual outside the family. We may need to hold a hand or to put an arm round a person who is in deep distress and give them the same kind of non-verbal assurance which a mother can give to her child. Nevertheless, even a mother who is comforting a child must remain in control. We must remain close but at the same time capable of taking a detached view of what is going on.

Difficult patients and difficult staff

A well organized network of care will deal with most of the problems which emerge with sufficient success for morale to be maintained among patients, families and staff for most of the time, but there are some situations of particular difficulty. The person whose insecurity causes him to panic, or cling or make angry and unreasonable demands is likely to be labelled as 'attention seeking'. This label may be justified, but it will only make the person more insecure if we get angry in return. If we recognize the underlying reason for such behaviour we shall usually end up supporting the person in the manner which suits him best. For some a firm line which says, 'I know what I'm doing and you're going to learn to trust me' is best; for others a full explanation of the nature of the treatments which are being prescribed, and for others positive reassurance will be needed. In all cases a listening ear and the opportunity to express feelings are prerequisites to successful care.

We shall often meet bravado in the compulsively self-reliant person who has never trusted anybody but himself—an attitude which often reflects deep-seated insecurity which may have been present from childhood. Such people need to believe that it is they who control us and not we who control them.

It is hard for a self-reliant person to accept the restrictions of illness and it often helps to show him that you realize how hard it is by discussing the problem. Staff members of a controlling disposition are likely to get at odds with this type of person. The doctor or nurse may be provoked to make disproportionate use of his or her power and in the end nobody emerges with credit. The care of the self-reliant requires patience, flexibility and not a little humility.

Paradoxically, it is often those who are most afraid of dying who demand euthanasia. They seem to be saying, 'Since I cannot avert the thing that I dread I will at least control it by choosing it for myself.' Again, the basic problem is lack of trust. Sometimes requests for euthanasia are reasonable requests for a way out of intolerable pain or physical distress. In such circumstances the obvious answer is to provide proper care so that the distress is relieved. Likewise, the relief of psychological distress will usually bring about a change in attitude to euthanasia. Among those who do not change their minds one often has the feeling that if one said, 'Do you want it now?' the patient would reply, 'No, but I would like to have it available in case I need it.' Similarly, one sometimes meets a depressed patient who keeps the means of suicide to hand as a source of reassurance.

Despite the prominence given to recent debates on euthanasia it is rare for a patient with incurable cancer to commit suicide. Nevertheless, suicides do occasionally occur, and we should be aware of that risk when assessing the mental state of any severely agitated or depressed person. The question, 'Has it been so bad that you have wanted to kill yourself?' will nearly always get an honest answer and we should never be afraid to ask. Once the risk is recognized it is usually possible to provide the physical and emotional care which will remove it.

Family members are often afraid that revealing the facts of his illness to the patient will cause him to kill himself. They may even try to force us to agree to a policy of concealment. Such fears are usually unrealistic and reflect the family's own fears of the situation. It follows that we should respond, not by colluding with the family or by ignoring their wishes, but by exploring with them their feelings about the situation and giving them the emotional support which they need if they are to support the patient.

Finding time

Of all the problems which we are faced with in the care of the dying patient, the greatest and one of the commonest is lack of time, either because the illness is progressing rapidly or because we are ourselves over-committed. In the latter case it should be possible to call on the help of others: a busy family doctor, for instance, may find that a health visitor or district nurse can spend time talking with patient and family, local clergy can be asked to provide pastoral care, neighbours or friends or the members of various voluntary organizations can be involved (see also Chapter 11). The problem resolves ultimately into one of priorities. How important is the contribution which doctors and nurses can make to the conscious life of a dying man? How does this compare with the importance of other demands upon our time?

If it is the patient who lacks time or is caught in a mesh of fear, denial or depression it may still be possible to achieve a lot with the judicious use of drugs. Drugs such as diazepam 5 mg 4-hourly are usually safe and often effective. If a more powerful agent is needed, a phenothiazine such as chlorpromazine 12·5–25 mg 4- to 6-hourly will reduce agitation. This has the advantage that phenothiazines potentiate the analgesic effects of morphine or diamorphine and can conveniently be added as a syrup to the narcotic mixture (see Chapter 5).

For the depressed patient who is inaccessible because he 'has given up' or who is failing to respond to our efforts to help, tricyclic antidepressants such as amitriptyline (which also help to reduce anxiety) 25 mg three times daily or 50–75 mg at night will often make life worth living. But we should expect to have to wait five to ten days for these drugs to become fully effective. The monoamine oxidase inhibitors should not be prescribed because they are incompatible with opiates and many of the other drugs which are likely to be needed in the terminal stage. On the other hand I have known a few cancer patients with psychotic levels of depression and psychomotor retardation who failed to respond to tricyclic antidepressants but made a rapid response to modified electric convulsive therapy.

The use of morphine and diamorphine is discussed elsewhere (Chapter 5) but it is worth noting at this point that they are themselves tranquillizers and are particularly effective when unpleasant physical symptoms are producing distress. Patients who are in severe physical distress are unlikely to make progress in tackling the psychological implications of their situation. But drugs should never be used as a substitute for personal attention and support. Drugs are not a way of relieving the care-givers of the responsibility of caring or of providing us with a 'happy ending' by 'knocking the patient out' ('she's asking questions—double the Largactil'). It is rarely necessary to render a patient unconscious in order to relieve distress, although many patients will become drowsy and at times a little confused in the last few hours or days of life.

Grief and the family

The use of drugs is much more controversial when we come to consider the needs of the relatives. As long as the patient is alive, they need to remain fully competent and to support the patient; clearly medication should be kept to a minimum. We should also be wary of using drugs after bereavement. Grief needs to be expressed and clinical experience suggests that drugs inhibit such expression. There are no grounds for prescribing tranquillizers or antidepressants to bereaved relatives as a routine. Such drugs should be reserved for the potentially suicidal and for those who, despite all efforts to help, remain in states of chronic agitation or depression for abnormally long periods.

The health of the newly bereaved is at risk in a number of ways, and the value of bereavement visiting has been established in at least three well conducted studies (Gerber *et al.*, 1975; Parkes, 1977; B. Raphael personal communication). Some families and some individuals within families are at greater risk than others.

Vulnerability

At St Christopher's Hospice we have identified as needing support in bereavement members of one family in four by using a screening procedure derived from the Harvard Bereavement Study (Parkes, 1976). There is evidence from our follow-up studies that these individuals are at greater risk than members of other families (to a statistically significant degree) but the results are not so clear-cut that we can say for sure that others should *not* be followed up.

Whether the screening procedure is used as a means of deciding who should be visited by a counsellor or simply as a way of alerting counsellors to the need to give rather more support to some than to others, it is suggested that attempts should be made to assess the risk to the person most affected by the patient's death whenever sufficient evidence is available.

The following people were found to be at special risk after bereavement:

1. Persons of low socioeconomic status.
2. Housewives without employment outside the house.
3. Those with young children at home (who may themselves be at risk).
4. Those without a supportive family or with a family who actively discourage the expression of grief.
5. Those who show a strong tendency to cling to the patient before his death and/or to pine intensely for him afterwards.
6. Those who express strong feelings of anger or bitterness before or after the patient's death.
7. Those who express strong feelings of self-reproach.

All these criteria can be assessed in about 90 per cent of the families of patients who die at St Christopher's Hospice. Other evidence of risk may emerge in a few cases. For instance, we may occasionally learn that a family member has a history of previous suicidal threats or psychiatric illness. Even if none of these criteria is satisfied, it should always be possible for staff members to request a follow-up visit although this is based on nothing more than a hunch.

It is still uncertain whether a formal screening procedure is necessary in order to identify those at risk. We have chosen not to submit bereaved family members to any form of questioning, but we use a standard assessment form which is completed by nurses or other professional staff who have become acquainted with the patient's family. The form refers to the key person thought to be most affected by the bereavement. It has been shown to have predictive validity. We follow up anyone scoring 19 or more on the form or rated 4 or 5 on question H. Any assessment of this kind must be treated as highly confidential and it is particularly important to avoid stigmatizing the bereaved people who are visited or creating problems by giving people the impression that they are expected to collapse under the strain of bereavement.

CONFIDENTIAL   Case Note

Name of patient   Age   Number:
(surname first in capitals)

Date of admission   Date of death:

Surname of   First
key person   Name:
Address: Telephone:

Relationship to patient   O.P.   Yes/No

Do you think key person would object to follow up?   Yes/No/Not known

Staff member(s) most closely involved:

Other family members in need of help:

Comments (include details of help already being given):

FSP   Signed: p.t.o.

Questionnaire (Ring one item in each section. Leave blank if not known):   CONFIDENTIAL

.... Tick here if key person not well enough known to enable these questions to be answered.

A.	B.	C.	D.	E.
Children under 14 at home	**Occupation of principal wage earner of key person's family****	**Employment of K.P. outside home**	**Clinging or pining**	**Anger**
0. None	1. Profes. & Exec.	0. Works F.T.	1. Never	1. None (or normal)
1. One	2. Semi-profes.	1. Works P/T	2. Seldom	2. Mild irritation
2. Two	3. Office & clerical	3. Retired	3. Moderate	3. Moderate—occasional outbursts
3. Three	4. Skilled manual	4. Housewife only	4. Frequent	4. Severe—spoiling relationships
4. Four	5. Semi-skilled manual	5. Unemployed	5. Constant	5. Extreme—always bitter
5. Five or more	6. Unskilled manual		6. Constant intense	
	** If in doubt, guess.			

F.	G.	H.
Self-reproach	**Relationship now**	**How will key person cope?** *
1. None	0. Close intimate relat. with another	1. **Well.** Normal grief and recovery without special help.
2. Mild vague & general	2. Warm supportive family permitting expression of feeling	2. **Fair,** probably get by without special help.
3. Moderate—some clear self-reproach	3. Family supportive but live at distance	3. **Doubtful,** may need special help.
4. Severe—preoc. self blame	4. Doubtful	4. **Badly,** requires special help.
5. Extreme—major problem	5. None of these	5. **Very badly,** requires urgent help.
		* All scoring 4 5 on H will be followed up.

Fig. 4.1. 'Key person' card.

Counselling the bereaved—early stage

The visiting should be low in profile and visitors should aim to reassure. We try to send someone already known to the family, such as a nurse, social worker or chaplain; if no suitable person is available, an experienced volunteer will be asked to call. The volunteers have been selected by the Hospice's volunteer organizer and, with close supervision and support from the social workers, they soon become more 'expert' at bereavement visiting than many of the professionals.

The initial visit is usually made 10–14 days after death. By this time the family, who have usually flocked round during the week of the funeral, have dispersed and the bereaved have come through the initial stage of shock or numbness. Grief is at its height and someone who calls at this time will usually find the bereaved glad of the opportunity to talk. Although the visitors have been warned never to press themselves on any person who seems reluctant to see them, it is almost unheard of for them to be treated as intruders. The visitor will almost always be told, 'You are the first person I've been able to talk to like this.' Bereaved people today often seem afraid of expressing their grief to their family for fear of upsetting them. Their friends, they think, will drop them if they embarrass them by crying; and the professionals, be they doctors, lawyers or bank managers, are thought to be too busy. Consequently, the visitor who has called 'Because I know what it is like and I thought you might like to talk about it' will be meeting an important need.

Apart from permitting the expression of grief and, in most cases, reassuring the bereaved that the violent emotions and physical sensations they are experiencing are normal, the visitor is able to assess the need for additional support. He or she can find out how much reliance the bereaved can place upon other family members and how many others rely on them. Some idea can also be obtained of the ways in which others are reacting to the loss and whether any of them are likely to need help. If there are health problems or there seems to be any danger of suicide, the visitor should urge the bereaved to obtain medical help and they should themselves report without delay to the doctor in charge of the visiting scheme so that he can contact the family doctor.

The help of social workers, lawyers, clergy and others may be needed. The initial visit may reveal that full support is already being provided and no further visits will be needed but in most cases several further visits will be necessary if only to ensure that the support which was anticipated is being given.

Counselling the bereaved—later stage

The grief of bereavement usually follows the pattern described on page 50. As the intensity and frequency of the pangs of grief grow less a different set of problems emerge. At this time it is more likely that the bereaved will need permission to stop grieving rather than to express grief. They may need to be helped to find new opportunities for personal development. It takes courage to recommit oneself in a world in which one has suffered a great loss. The bereaved have discovered that grief is the price they pay for love and they hesitate to pay that price again. And yet in time they may also find that they have survived the pain of grief and that death has left them more willing to recognize the full range of meanings—good and bad—which life offers to us.

I make no apology for these high-sounding words for they reflect my admiration for many of the people who have shared their grief with me. Just as close relationships with the dying help to reduce our fears of death, so counselling the bereaved makes it easier to recognize bereavement as an acceptable part of life.

Every bereavement is different and we can never know how a person will emerge. People who deny the need to grieve by filling their lives with activities or by getting rid of all reminders of the lost person are only storing up trouble. In this instance it is important to reassure them that it is safe to grieve and to seek for 'linking objects'—mementoes, photographs and the like—which help to trigger repressed grief. Once grief has been expressed it will tend to follow a more normal course.

Anger and guilt

The expression of anger or guilt after bereavement is one of the most difficult problems. At this stage it is too late to say, 'I'm sorry', and the bereaved are sometimes tempted to punish themselves or those around them by endless and embittered grieving ('grief' and 'aggrieved' have a common origin). Yet many bereaved people discover ways of expressing their discontent which are creative rather than destructive (St Christopher's Hospice is itself the consequence of one such creative endeavour). The role of the counsellor is to provide a sounding board, a patient and understanding person who will accept the contradictions of ambivalence without criticism or rejection. But the function of the sounding board is not just to absorb; when the right note is struck it can resound and respond with encouragement and hope. The bereavement counsellor is not passive but alert to all that is passing and ready to give praise and comfort when it is due.

Suicide

The importance of assessing suicidal risk cannot be over-stressed and we should never hesitate to ask direct questions on this topic. Bereavement is one of the commonest causes of suicide, and much needless loss of life could be prevented if we faced up to the implications of this fact.

Several studies have shown that the majority of suicidal people talk about their plans before a suicidal attempt is made. The person who is a serious suicidal risk may not mention the fact unless directly questioned but will then be found to have a well thought out plan. On the other hand remarks such as, 'I wouldn't care if I died tomorrow' seldom indicate a true suicidal intent.

Those tempted to suicide are often isolated from their families and it is important to draw in the support of someone who can keep a close eye on them until the danger is past. In some cases the family doctor may need to arrange admission to psychiatric care, in others he may decide that the situation can be contained at home. In either case he will be well advised to encourage visitors to continue their support. Given the choice between taking an overdose and phoning the friend who has left a telephone number 'which you can ring at any time if things get unbearable', the potential suicide will often choose the latter course.

Withdrawal from life

For those who lack confidence to begin again, either because they have always had a low opinion of themselves or because there is little inducement to look forward, it is tempting to use grief as an excuse to withdraw from life. In such cases the counsellor may be misused as a means of validating this withdrawal ('You understand how much I loved him, you tell them that I am sick'). Like the physically disabled patient who clings on to the 'sick role' after the illness is past, so the mourner may demand endorsement of the 'mourning role'.

Those who are particularly lonely or lacking in confidence can easily come to rely too much on the visitor. In such cases the time will come for the counsellor to prepare a plan for his or her own withdrawal. This is not done in an abrupt or rejecting way but the usual rule of medical care (the sicker the patient the more care he gets) must be reversed. Continued support becomes conditional upon the bereaved person moving towards the accomplishment of a new set of goals. It sounds brutal to say 'Ring me again when you have got a job', but this is sometimes necessary and, provided our expectations are not unrealistic, will usually produce results. Often a small initial success leads to a greater one. If this policy is adopted, the danger of the bereaved becoming perpetually dependent on the counsellor is negligible.

The care-givers

In the brief compass of this chapter it has been impossible to do more than touch on the range of problems which are as numerous and as varied as the people who suffer them. In offering guidelines, I have inevitably over-simplified in the interests of clarity. Not all the people we set out to help will benefit from our ministrations and we must be prepared to admit and understand our own failures.

The risk of failure should not deter us from trying. There is no such thing as a 'hopeless case' and no excuse for ignoring the psychological needs of the dying and the bereaved. If we accept that fact we should provide as wide a range as possible of skilled people to meet these needs. In suggesting that there is a place for volunteers and others with little training in psychological medicine, I do not mean to infer that more sophisticated approaches are never needed. The needs of the dying and the bereaved will sometimes tax the skills of the most experienced social workers and psychiatrists and it is important that these are available as a source of additional help.

Support to the supporters

The capacity of the care-givers to cope with the emotional needs of patients and families is fostered by a support system which encourages them to put into words and share with each other their perceptions of the life situations which they encounter. The support group should be sufficiently open with each other for it to be possible for them to talk, not only about the emotional problems of the patients and families whom they are trying to help but also about the feelings which these people evoke in themselves. A well functioning support group will know when one of its members is becoming too closely involved and will move at once to support him or her—either by taking over some of the care or by pointing out what the care-giver is doing in the hope that, with insight, he or she will behave more appropriately. Similarly, a group may help one of its members to understand why a particular patient angers others or makes them feel guilty; in doing so, the group will help him to take a more objective view of a painful situation.

It is, of course, essential for group members to be able to trust each other and a support group is no place for scoring points off each other or undermining confidence. The senior member of the group carries particular responsibility for ensuring that the group is truly supportive and, within a particular institution, it is likely that the leaders will need their own support group.

There will always be some who, for one reason or another, are not adequately helped by their own work team. Hierarchical struggles within the team or fear of censure from above may reduce the effectiveness of a support group. For this reason it is important to ensure that there are a number of alternative sources of support available to staff who are working in emotionally charged situations. The visiting psychiatrist has an important role to play here, but not everyone wants to talk to a psychiatrist; a range of nurse advisers, visiting clergy, social workers and others should be accessible and able to provide individual or group support. A terminal care unit should be a community—a network in which nobody feels isolated.

Much support will be informal and take place outside formal staff meetings. There are no rigid roles; at times we shall be care-givers and at other times cared-for. The senior staff must keep a close watch for sources of strain within a particular part of the organization—a spate of deaths on one ward, the absence on leave of a key member of staff, the effects of an influenza epidemic on staffing levels or the approaching death of a favourite patient should all alert the seniors to give extra support to a particular part of the system. It is essential to have sufficient numbers and flexibility of staff to ensure that this support is available.

The psychiatrist has a particular responsibility as the person to whom the most difficult or intractable problems can be referred. My own experience at St Christopher's Hospice indicates that these cases are comparatively few (of the order of 10–15 per cent). Much more important is the role of the psychiatrist as a support to the front-line care-givers. He should play a part in organizing and maintaining a high standard of psychosocial care; teaching the medical and nursing staff, consulting with staff about the patients and family members under their care and, at times, providing individual support to staff members who have problems of their own (although it is probably advisable to refer them to other places if long-term therapy is required).

The sharing of information within the care-giving team is a necessary activity in any therapeutic community in which the responsibility for care is shared by a number of people. It implies that the team as a whole will exercise professional standards of discretion and will not gossip outside the work group or otherwise misuse the information at their disposal. Within the team a free and frequent interchange of ideas and observations should be encouraged. I have been repeatedly impressed by the way in which a group of nurses on a ward can piece together the information which each of them has picked up in day-to-day interaction with a family to make a picture of the whole which immediately explains why a particular patient or family member is in difficulties. Apart from the value of this exercise to the person they are trying to help the sharing of information in this way alerts the staff to the importance of listening.

Terminal care is a matter of human relationships. There are skills to be learned and insights which can be gained from reading books but the challenge and the reward of terminal care arises from the fact that it demands that we use the whole of ourselves to relate to fellow human beings who are in trouble. This can only be learned by experience in a community in which relationships are valued and fostered.

' "Mourning is not forgetting," he said gently, his helplessness vanishing and his voice becoming wise. "It is an undoing. Every minute tie has to be untied and something permanent and valuable recovered and assimilated from the knot. The end is gain, of course. Blessed are they that mourn, for they shall be made strong, in fact. But the process is like all other human births, painful and long and dangerous." '

Allingham, 1957

References

ALLINGHAM, Margery (1957). *The Tiger in the Smoke*. Penguin; Harmondsworth, Middx.

CANNON, W. B. (1929). *Bodily Changes in Pain, Hunger, Fear and Rage*. Appleton; London and New York.

CASSELL, E. (1974). Dying in a technological society. In: *Death Inside Out*, p. 43. Ed. by P. Steinfels and R. M. Veatch. Harper & Row; New York.

GERBER, I., WIENER, A., BATTIN, D. and ARKIN, A. (1975). Brief therapy to the aged bereaved. Chapter 27 in: *Bereavement: Its Psychosocial Aspects*. Ed. by B. Schoenberg *et al*. Columbia University Press; New York.

GLICK, I. O., WEISS, R. S. and PARKES, C. M. (1974). *The First Year of Bereavement*. Wiley; New York.

NIGHTINGALE, F. (1946) *The Art of Nursing*. Claud Morris, London.

PARKES, C. M. (1972a). *Bereavement: Studies of Grief in Adult Life*. Tavistock and Pelican; London. International Universities Press; New York.

PARKES, C. M. (1972b). Accuracy of predictions of survival in later stages of cancer. *British Medical Journal* 2, 29.

PARKES, C. M. (1973). Attachment and autonomy at the end of life. In: *Support, Innovation and Autonomy*, pp. 151–166. Ed. by R. Gosling. Tavistock; London.

PARKES, C. M. (1976). Determinants of outcome following bereavement. *Omega* 6, 303.

PARKES, C. M. (1977). Evaluation of family care in terminal illness. In: *The Family and Death: Social Work Perspectives*. Ed. by E. R. Pritchard, J. Collard, B. A. Orcutt, A. H. Kutscher, I. Seeland and N. Lefkowitz. Columbia University Press; New York.

PARKES, C. M. (1978). Home or Hospital? Patterns of care for the terminally ill cancer patient as seen by surviving spouses. *Journal of the Royal College of General Practitioners*, **28**, 19–30.

RAPHAEL, B. (1977) Personal Communication.

ROSS, E. K. (1970). *On Death and Dying*. Tavistock; London.

SCHULTZ, R. and ADERMAN, D. (1974). Clinical research and the stages of dying. *Omega* 5, 137.

WEISMAN, A. D. and WORDEN, J. (1975). Psychosocial analysis of cancer deaths. *Omega* 6, 61.

5

Relief of Pain

Robert G. Twycross

Editorial note

'Unrelieved, relievable distress'

> 'Pain is the resultant of the conflict between the stimulus and the whole individual.'
> Leriche, 1939

> 'Although I arrived with an initial resistance to continual contact with the dying patient, the actual experience was quite different from what I had expected. Instead of a terminal care or "death house" environment with cachetic, narcotized, bedridden, depressed patients, I found an active community of patients, staff, families and children of staff and patients.'
> Liegner, 1975

People of many professions are involved with patients needing terminal care, practising a combination of the science and art of medicine in different settings. In the past few decades a great deal has been learned of both, and this knowledge is being spread in writing and at many conferences;* the problem of relieving distress is at last receiving the attention it deserves.

Yet we continue to meet patients who give us histories of weeks and months of unrelieved pain, anorexia, vomiting, incontinence and other forms of physical distress. Sometimes it appears that no attempt has been made to relieve them. A professor of nursing who has done extensive research in the United States writes: 'If most nurses carry the notion that pain is usual with cancer, then one must assume that many nurses believe that pain and cancer always go hand in hand (as does the public at large)' (Benoliel, 1974).

The knowledge that only 50 per cent of cancer patients are likely to have pain is discussed below, but the studies of Hinton (1963), Parkes (1977) and Rees (1972) and the Royal College of Nursing resolution (p. 151) show that no-one can be complacent about the proportion of that 50 per cent whose pain remains uncontrolled. There is every hope that in the future we shall develop better and more rational therapy but with the tools we now possess no patient should suffer from inept treatment. Robbie describes the nerve blocks and other procedures commonly used at earlier stages of the disease but occasionally called on for patients who are terminally ill.

Twycross's chapter summarizes our present state of knowledge concerning the drugs

---

*See, for example, the Annual Conference of the Marie Curie Memorial Foundation, St Christopher's Annual Therapeutics Conference, St Joseph's half-day meetings and many others in the United Kingdom; many conferences are held in the United States of America. A leaflet, 'Drug Control of Common Symptoms' has proved popular and useful (*World Medicine*, 1978). It is available from St Christopher's and St Joseph's Hospices.

available for the control of terminal pain and the painstaking research which has gone into it. Baines presents a clear and practical guide to the control of the many symptoms, other than pain, which may burden these patients, and she leads us continually to seek for the cause of these symptoms—topics already discussed in Chapters 2 and 3. We should be replacing empirical and sometimes blunderbuss therapy with more finely honed tools. The foundations for this work are at last being laid, but in the meantime knowledge is sufficiently established for there to be no longer any excuse for unrelieved, terminal physical distress.

References

BENOLIEL, J. Q. (1974). *The Patient in Pain: New Concepts.* American Cancer Society; New York.
HINTON, J. M. (1963). The physical and mental distress of the dying. *Quarterly Journal of Medicine N.S.* **32**, 1.
LIEGNER, L. (1975). St. Christopher's Hospice 1974: care of the dying patient. *Journal of the American Medical Association* **234**, 1047.
LERICHE, R. (1939) *The Surgery of Pain.* Translated and edited by A. Young, Bailliére Tindall and Cox, London.
PARKES, C. M. (1977). Evaluation of family care in terminal illness. In: *The Family and Death.* Ed. by E. R. Pritchard, J. Collard, B. A. Orcutt, A. H. Kutscher, I. Seeland and N. Lefkowicz. Columbia University Press; New York.
REES, W. D. (1972). The distress of dying. *British Medical Journal* **2**, 105.

'Among the remedies which it has pleased Almighty God to give to man to relieve his sufferings, none is so universal and so efficacious as opium.'
    Thomas Sydenham, 1680

'He was far too humble and indeed, too experienced, to expect that the Almighty's more quixotic benefits should ever prove to be unadulterated jam.'
    Allingham, 1957

To many people, incurable cancer means a painful progressive illness ending in an agonizing death. In fact, possibly as many as 50 per cent of patients with advanced cancer have no pain at all or negligible discomfort at most; 40 per cent experience severe pain and the remaining 10 per cent mild to moderate pain (Turnbull, 1954; Aitken-Swan, 1959). At St Christopher's Hospice and similar institutions, the incidence of pain on admission is higher, in the region of 75 per cent. This is partly because unrelieved pain is a common reason for referral by general practitioners and partly because patients in pain are given priority among admissions. Recently published data (Parkes, 1977) indicate that the degree of success in relieving terminal pain is considerably greater in a specialized unit compared with general hospital (Fig. 5.1). If the level of success achieved in the former could be obtained more generally, the prospect for the patient with incurable cancer would be correspondingly enhanced.

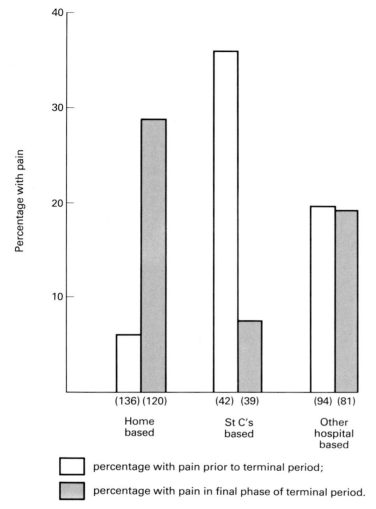

Fig. 5.1. Histogram showing percentage of patients with severe and mostly continuous pain in groups of patients with terminal cancer cared for at home, or at St Christopher's Hospice or in other hospitals. In those cared for by St Christopher's, although more of them experienced pain preterminally, the number with pain terminally (and after contact with the Hospice) is markedly less. Assessments were based on interview with the closest relative several months after the patient's death. Figures in parentheses refer to the number of patients interviewed.

The nature of pain

There are many reasons for failure to relieve pain (Hunt *et al.*, 1977) but perhaps one of the most important is a failure by doctors and nurses to appreciate fully that pain is not simply a physical sensation. It is, in fact, a dual phenomenon; one part being the perception of the sensation and the other the patient's emotional reaction to it. It follows that a person's pain threshold will vary according to mood and morale, and intensity of pain likewise. Attention must therefore be paid to non-pharmacological factors which modulate pain threshold as well as to the correct use of analgesic and other drugs (Table 5.1).

Death is probably the loneliest experience any of us will ever have to face. Most patients fear the process of dying—'Will it hurt?', 'Will I suffocate?' —and many fear death itself. Many of these fears will remain unspoken unless the patient is given the opportunity to express them. The doctor needs to give time and opportunity for the patient to talk about his progress or lack of it. Sometimes a patient needs 'permission to talk' and a question such as, 'Are you worried about yourself?' may enable the patient to say or ask what he desperately wishes to but feels unable to because 'Doctor hasn't got time to stop and talk' or 'Doctor is too busy to be concerned with my problems'. These important questions are discussed more fully in Chapters 1, 4 and 10.

Table 5.1   Factors which modify pain threshold

Discomfort Insomnia Fatigue Anxiety Fear Anger Sadness Depression Mental isolation Introversion (Past experience)	THRESHOLD LOWERED	Relief of symptoms Sleep Rest Sympathy Understanding Diversion Elevation of mood Analgesics Anxiolytics Antidepressants	THRESHOLD RAISED

Sir David Smithers, sometime Director of Radiotherapy Department, Royal Marsden Hospital, made it a rule that his registrar should visit terminally ill patients each day. Moreover, he said that, however brilliant a clinical pharmacologist a doctor may be, if he has no time for chat, he knows nothing about terminal care (Smithers, 1973). In this context, chat means 'patient chat' while the doctor listens. Although sometimes this is very demanding of both time and emotion, the benefits are considerable. To quote from the experience of one group of general practitioners: 'As the doctor–patient relationship improved, many doctors found they could reduce the drugs. As the true diagnosis of the patient's pain became clear and the patient was helped to deal with the pain of dying, there was less need for sedatives, tranquillizers and analgesics' (Harte, J. D., 1975, personal communication).

Assessment of pain

A diagnosis of cancer does not necessarily mean that the malignant process is the cause of the pain. As always, diagnosis must precede treatment. Constipation, peptic ulcer, pressure sores, cystitis and musculoskeletal disorders may be responsible, and all are conditions which benefit from more specific treatment. When the cancer is responsible, it is important to consider the exact cause of the pain, as treatment may differ if it is due to involvement of bone or nerve compression rather than local soft tissue infiltration.

Site and intensity

Pain may be limited to one site or be multifocal. Each site where pain is felt should be recorded. A body image may be of value here (Fig. 5.2). It acts as a baseline for future reference and helps in the consideration of underlying

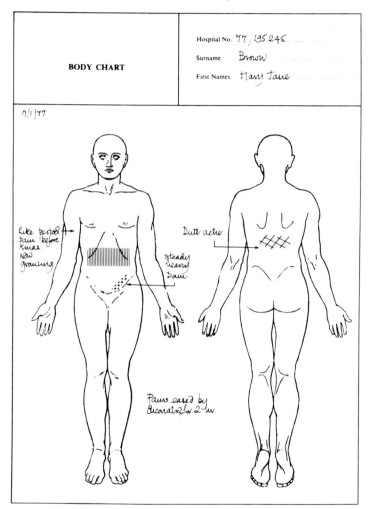

Fig. 5.2. Body image for recording sites of pain and related data.

mechanisms. Intensity is assessed on the basis of both the patient's description of the pain—'mild', 'moderate', 'severe'—and the success or failure of past medication (Table 5.2). Detailed assessment is difficult when pain is overwhelming and one is faced with a distressed, exhausted patient who says or implies 'It's all pain, doctor'. This together with a catalogue of failed remedies

Table 5.2   Clinical classification of pain intensity

Intensity	Fails to respond to	Relieved by
Mild		Non-narcotic analgesics aspirin paracetamol
Moderate	Non-narcotic analgesics	Weak narcotic analgesics codeine dihydrocodeine dextropropoxyphene pentazocine pethidine
Severe	Weak narcotic analgesics	Intermediate strength narcotics dipipanone papaveretum
Very severe	Intermediate strength narcotics	Potent narcotic analgesics morphine diamorphine levorphanol phenazocine (methadone)
Overwhelming	Potent narcotic analgesics alone	Potent analgesics + sedative–anxiolytic diazepam chlorpromazine (methotrimeprazine)

is, however, sufficient to allow treatment with a potent analgesic in combination with chlorpromazine or diazepam.

Quality

Patients often find it difficult to describe the quality of pain, though if adjectives are used, or agreed with, it helps in deciding the mechanism of the pain (Duboisson and Melzack, 1976). 'Like raving toothache' or 'sharp, shooting pain, especially on movement' suggest nerve compression and will influence the course of treatment should analgesics alone fail to relieve.

A 68-year-old man with disseminated carcinoma of the prostate was admitted with pain in the right knee. The pain was 'like pins and needles but hundreds of times worse'. This information, coupled with wasting of the ipsilateral quadriceps femoris, suggested involvement of the right femoral nerve. Accordingly, the analgesic regimen was left unaltered and prednisolone (see p. 90) prescribed. This resulted in complete relief within a few days.

Variation

Intensity of pain may vary considerably during the day. There are undoubtedly several reasons for this (Glynn et al., 1976) but the use of medication which eases pain for an hour or two is often a major factor. Such data should be carefully recorded because the information afforded helps in the choice of analgesic, dose and frequency of administration. In some patients, pain is minimal at rest but intolerable on movement or when walking. Relationship to micturition, defaecation, eating, breathing, coughing or posture should also be noted.

A 4-year-old child with an inoperable pontine glioma experienced increasing pain in the head and occipital region. She lay flat all the time because elevation of the head caused a marked increase in pain. With this history it was necessary to postulate a local source of pain (possibly caused by post-radiation meningeal adhesions) in addition to the diffuse headache of secondary hydrocephalus (which would have been helped by a more erect posture). The diffuse pain was relieved by small regular doses of an opiate but not until she was transferred to a bed which allowed elevation of the head, neck and trunk in unison was it possible for the child to sit up without pain. Subsequently, it became possible to transfer the child from bed to a high-backed reclining chair, and even to lift her on to her mother's lap. This suggested that some of the pain had been caused by spasm of the neck muscles, and that the confidence engendered by the ability to sit up in bed allowed additional manoeuvres to be undertaken without pain.

Reassessment

The probability of the initial prescription being inadequate increases with the intensity of pain. Patients should therefore be reassessed within hours if the pain is overwhelming, or after 1 or 2 days if severe or moderate. If troublesome or unacceptable side-effects result, treatment may need to be modified. In addition, the relief of the major pain may allow a second, less severe, pain to become apparent.

An 85-year-old man with carcinoma of the prostate and pain in the right femur caused by metastatic tumour was treated with aspirin and an opiate. Casual questioning the next day indicated that, although less severe, he was still in pain. Further questioning revealed that the site of pain was now retrosternal and epigastric; he had no femoral pain at all. The dose of the opiate was, therefore, left unaltered, and the prescription of an antacid resulted in complete relief.

General principles

Acute (transient) and chronic (persistent) pain are as different from one another as acute and chronic renal failure. It is all too easy for a doctor to forget this when, in all probability, he has no personal experience of chronic pain. His understanding of pain is usually taken from his own experience of acute pain—toothache, headache, bruise or sprain—all of which pass relatively quickly. On the other hand, chronic pain is a situation rather than an event and it:

1. is impossible to predict when it will end;
2. usually gets worse rather than better;
3. lacks positive meaning;
4. frequently expands to occupy the patient's whole attention; and when this happens, life is no longer worth living.

The differences between acute and chronic pain are reflected in the way analgesics are administered in the two situations (Table 5.3). Pain is a potent 'algesic', and to allow the pain to re-emerge before administering the next dose

Table 5.3   Comparison of analgesic use in acute and chronic pain

	Acute	Chronic
Aim	Pain relief	Pain relief
Sedation	Often desirable	Usually undesirable
Desired duration of effect	2–4 hours	As long as possible
Timing	As required (on demand)	Regularly (in anticipation)
Dose	Usually standard	Individually determined
Route	Injection	By mouth
Adjuvant medication	Uncommon	Common

not only causes unnecessary suffering but encourages tolerance. Accordingly, '4-hourly as required' has no place in the treatment of persistent pain. Whatever its aetiology, *chronic pain requires regular preventive therapy*. The aim is to titrate the level of analgesia against the patient's pain, gradually increasing the dose until the patient is pain-free. The next dose is given before the effect of the previous one has worn off and, therefore, before the patient may think it necessary. It is thus possible to erase the memory and fear of pain. As patients do not like constantly taking tablets or receiving injections, a 4-hourly interval between doses should be regarded as the norm, though occasionally a shorter period may be necessary. Many patients do not require a dose at 2 a.m., though, if necessary, a patient should be wakened to take it rather than let him wake later complaining of pain.

As already mentioned, doses should be determined on an individual basis; the right dose of any analgesic is that which gives adequate relief for at least 3 and preferably 4 or more hours. Patients will usually accept two, sometimes three, analgesic tablets per administration, together with additional medication; four or more tablets of the same preparation are generally not acceptable. Thus, if two tablets are not adequate, the patient should be transferred to a more potent alternative. In many cases this will be a narcotic analgesic. The considerable between-patient variation with respect to effective analgesic dose and the fact that administration is by mouth rather than by injection means that 'maximum' or 'recommended' doses, derived mainly from postoperative parenteral single-dose studies, are not applicable to the treatment of pain in advanced cancer.

Choice of analgesic

Mild pain

Mild pain, by definition, responds to aspirin or paracetamol. These are available in soluble and non-soluble forms both 'over the counter' and on prescription. If unsupervised, patients tend to take these preparations not more than three times a day which results in a 'switchback' effect. When this occurs, patients should be advised to take medication more frequently, either 4- or 6-hourly, in order to anticipate and prevent the re-emergence of pain.

Many patients can tolerate up to 1200 mg of aspirin 4-hourly, obtaining relief denied to them with the more usual 600 mg dose. If a higher dose is recommended, the problem of patient compliance can be overcome by using a soluble form which converts four tablets into one drink, or by prescribing a

Table 5.4   Useful preparations of aspirin

Preparation	Aspirin content per tablet (mg)	Mode of administration	Interval between doses (hours)
Aspirin	300	Swallow whole	4
Soluble aspirin	300	Dissolve in water	4
Aspirin–glycine (Paynocil)	600	Dissolve on tongue	4
Enteric-coated aspirin (Nu-seals)	325, 650	Swallow whole	8
Microencapsulated aspirin (Levius)	500	Swallow whole	8
Aloxiprin (aluminium polyoxoaspirin; Palaprin Forte)	500	Dissolve in water suck, chew or swallow whole	4

preparation such as Paynocil (Table 5.4). If dyspepsia or gastrointestinal bleeding is a problem, enteric-coated aspirin or aloxiprin may be tried. The size of the former preparation tends, however, to reduce its usefulness in advanced cancer (though, in arthritis, the more sustained blood level reaching a maximum after about 8 hours means that a bedtime dose helps to alleviate morning stiffness). Benorylate, an ester of aspirin and paracetamol which needs only to be administered two or three times a day, cannot be recommended for routine use because of the considerably greater cost of a week's average treatment.

Moderate pain

When aspirin or paracetamol fail to relieve, weak narcotic analgesics, such as codeine, dihydrocodeine (DHC) and dextropropoxyphene, should be used either alone or in combination with aspirin or paracetamol (Table 5.5). It is generally stated that DHC is one-third, and codeine one-sixth as potent as morphine. These are almost certainly over-optimistic estimates; in cancer pain, DHC is approximately one-sixth as potent as morphine (Seed *et al.*, 1958), and codeine one-twelfth (Houde, Wallenstein and Beaver, 1965). Although DHC is more potent than codeine, any difference between them is reduced by the constraints of tablet size. DHC is said to be less constipating than codeine.

Dextropropoxyphene continues to enjoy considerable vogue. In Great Britain, it is generally used in combination with paracetamol (Distalgesic), whereas in the United States it is used both alone (Darvon) and in combination (Darvon-Co). The popularity appears to result from several factors, including a widespread belief in its efficacy, not wholly supported by evidence from clinical trials (Miller, Feingold and Paxinos, 1970) and the fact that, unlike aspirin and aspirin-compound tablets, dextropropoxyphene is available only on prescription. In other words, it will not have been tried and found wanting by the patient prior to prescription by the doctor, and will therefore be taken with a higher expectancy of success than a self-prescribed remedy. Until more evidence is forthcoming to show that it is superior to aspirin or

Table 5.5   Weak narcotic analgesic preparations

	Narcotic	Adjuvant	Proprietary preparation
Dextropropoxyphene 1	65	—	Doloxene
2	150	—	Depronal SA
+ aspirin 1	(50) *	500	Napsalgesic
2	(100) *	325	Dolasan
+ paracetamol	32·5	325	Distalgesic
Codeine phosphate	15, 30, 60	—	—
+ aspirin	8	500	Codis
+ paracetamol	8	500	Neurodyne Panadeine
Dihydrocodeine tartrate	30	—	DF 118
+ aspirin	10	300	Onadox-118
+ paracetamol	10	500	Paramol-118

* Weight refers to dextropropoxyphene *napsylate*; equivalent to 32·5 and 65 mg of hydrochloride, respectively.

paracetamol, either alone or in combination with codeine, its true place in therapeutics will continue to be uncertain.

Pentazocine—a partial agonist—and pethidine have little or no place in the treatment of chronic pain. By mouth, 50 mg of pentazocine is less potent than two tablets of codeine phosphate plus aspirin (Codis) or of dextro-propoxyphene plus paracetamol (Distalgesic) (Robbie and Samarasinghe, 1973). Furthermore, the proportion of patients experiencing nalorphine-like psychotomimetic side-effects (Wood *et al.*, 1974) is unacceptably high when there are safer alternatives. Although such side-effects tend to be dose-related, they have been observed after even small doses by mouth. Similarly, orally administered pethidine should not be regarded as a potent analgesic and, by injection, it acts only for some 2–3 hours (Marks and Sachar, 1973).

Severe pain

Papaveretum (Omnopon) and dipipanone are useful intermediates between the weak and the potent narcotic analgesics. Dipipanone is available only with cyclizine as Diconal, but there is no evidence that it causes more nausea than other narcotics (Dundee and Jones, 1968). Alternatively, a solution of opium (Nepenthe) may be used, with or without aspirin. Each 1 ml of undiluted Nepenthe contains the equivalent of about 12 mg of morphine (in terms of sulphate) and is usually supplied as a 10 per cent (1 ml in 10) or 20 per cent (2 ml in 10) solution in chloroform water; precipitation occurs when stronger solutions are dispensed.

Diamorphine and morphine are usually given in solution, and traditionally have been dispensed in a vehicle containing alcohol and syrup. Some patients, however, complain about the 'sickliness' of such mixtures, while others dislike the alcoholic 'bite'. It is recommended, therefore, that diamorphine and morphine be dispensed in chloroform water alone, the patient adding blackcurrant or other fruit juice if desired.* If dispensed with a phenothiazine, the incorporation of one of the flavoured proprietary syrups usually circumvents the need for additional flavouring. The use of local names, such as 'Brompton Cocktail', 'Haustus E' and 'Mist. Euphoria' to describe solutions of diamorphine or morphine (with or without cocaine) is to be discouraged, as it obscures the content not only from the patient but also from the prescribing doctor. As diamorphine in solution hydrolyses to O^6-monoacetylmorphine (O^6-MAM) and eventually to morphine, unused solutions should be discarded after 6 weeks (Twycross, 1974a). If dispensed with a phenothiazine, hydrolysis is accelerated and the shelf-life is reduced to about 2 weeks; however, as it is unusual to dispense quantities for more than this period, this is rarely a limiting factor.

The use of solutions gives considerable freedom in relation to dose. At St Christopher's Hospice, oral diamorphine was prescribed in quantities ranging from as little as 2·5 mg to as much as 90 mg in 10 ml (Fig. 5.3). If the latter

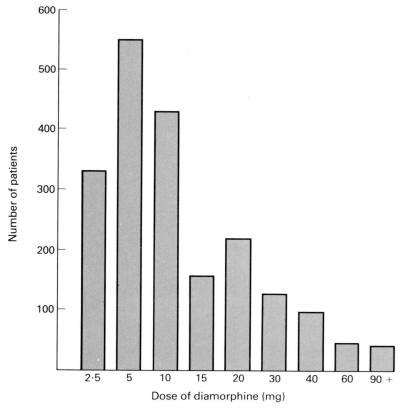

Fig. 5.3. Histogram of maximum 4-hourly doses of diamorphine given to 2000 patients admitted to St Christopher's Hospice, 1972–1975 inclusive.

* Or his alcohol of choice.—Ed.

proves ineffectual, medication is given by injection. Because diamorphine is more potent by injection than by mouth, it is conventional to halve the dose when changing to parenteral administration. Most patients, however, can be maintained on oral medication. The main indication for parenteral administration, apart from extreme debility, is intractable nausea and vomiting despite the prescription of an antiemetic. The need for injections may sometimes be avoided by the use of morphine suppositories. Several strengths are available ranging from 10 to 60 mg; morphine per rectum is equipotent with morphine by mouth. Proladone suppositories,* which contain 30 mg oxycodone pectinate, are also available. Each 30 mg suppository is equivalent to 20 mg morphine. After administration the oxycodone is slowly released from the pectin core over several hours. Thus one or two suppositories every 6 or 8 hours may be adequate. Alternatively, round-the-clock relief may be maintained by using Duromorph, a microcrystalline suspension of morphine, two or three times a day. It is available in capped vials each containing 70·4 mg morphine base in 1·1 ml (64 mg/ml).

Overwhelming pain

Extremely severe pain engenders fear and, if prolonged, results in physical exhaustion. It should be regarded as a medical emergency, and diamorphine with chlorpromazine or diazepam should be given by injection until the pain is controlled. The dose will depend on the patient's age, weight and previous medication. If the pain is not eased considerably, the initial injection may need to be both increased and repeated every 1 or 2 hours until relief is obtained. A 3- to 4-hourly regimen can then be determined, based on initial requirements. Once the pain is relieved, the patient may sleep for long periods until thoroughly rested. It is important to appreciate that the larger the effective analgesic dose the shorter will be its duration of action. When injections of more than 30 mg are needed, a 3-hour regimen may be necessary; with more than 60 mg, the interval may need to be even less. After control has been achieved and maintained for several days it may be possible to reduce the dose, extend the interval between administrations, or transfer the patient on to oral medication for continuing pain control.

Diamorphine or morphine?

In a trial involving nearly 700 patients at St Christopher's Hospice (Twycross, 1977), it was demonstrated that patients receiving individually determined doses of morphine by mouth fared as well as those receiving diamorphine (Fig. 5.4). After 2 weeks, if well enough, patients 'crossed' from one opiate to the other. The potency ratio for orally administered diamorphine and morphine was shown to be 1·5:1.

In a parallel study of urinary excretion of morphine in patients receiving diamorphine or morphine regularly, the results indicated that diamorphine is completely absorbed by the gastrointestinal tract but that morphine is only some two-thirds absorbed (Twycross, Fry and Wills, 1974). This finding suggests that the potency ratio of orally administered diamorphine and morphine merely reflects the alimentary absorption ratio of the two preparations. This

* This drug has been temporarily discontinued; morphine suppositories 15–30 mg 6-hourly may be used instead.

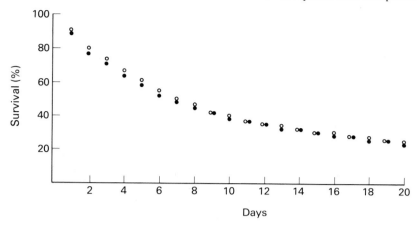

Fig. 5.4. Survival chart for 350 patients receiving oral diamorphine every 4 hours in individually determined doses (o) and 349 patients receiving morphine (●). Untoward side-effects and need for adjuvant medication were also similar.

accords with the view of Way, Young and Kemp (1965)—based largely on studies using organ homogenates from both animals and man—that diamorphine is so rapidly deacetylated *in vivo* to O^6-MAM and morphine that it has only a transient pharmacological action of its own even after intravenous injection, its effects being almost entirely mediated via its two biotransformation products.

On the other hand, when injections are necessary, the greater solubility of its hydrochloride (1 g in 1·6 ml) gives diamorphine an important practical advantage over morphine sulphate or hydrochloride (1 g in > 20 ml). This means that an injection of diamorphine hydrochloride, available as a freeze-dried pellet, will rarely need to exceed 0·1 ml in volume. Other morphine salts are, however, more soluble: tartrate twice, and acetate ten times more than the sulphate or hydrochloride (Martindale, 1977). Unfortunately, morphine acetate is unstable in solution and the resultant free morphine is practically insoluble in water. Similarly, although 100 mg of morphine tartrate in theory will dissolve in 1 ml, in practice it is generally less soluble due to contamination with an acid tartrate (Cooper, J. B., 1972, personal communication). Consequently, there is little advantage in its use.

To summarize, provided allowance is made for the difference in potency, morphine is satisfactory as a substitute for orally administered diamorphine. If injections are necessary, the greater solubility of its hydrochloride gives diamorphine an important practical advantage over morphine, especially when large doses are required.

Alternatives to diamorphine and morphine

Both levorphanol (Dromoran) and phenazocine (Narphen) are approximately three times more potent than diamorphine on a weight-for-weight basis. Moreover, both have a more prolonged plasma half-life than diamorphine and morphine and frequently can be given 6-, sometimes 8-hourly. This is an advantage if a 4-hourly regimen is impractical or inconvenient. Phenazocine is also effective sublingually and, if the patient is able to tolerate the bitter taste, its use in this way may circumvent the need for injections in patients with severe dysphagia. Methadone, which has a plasma half-life of more than 70 hours (Verebely et al., 1975) may also be useful in these circumstances though, because of the danger of accumulation, should not be used in very ill or elderly patients.

Dextromoramide (Palfium) is prescribed by many doctors as an alternative to diamorphine or morphine and, for some patients, seems to be a satisfactory substitute. By mouth it is comparable to diamorphine on a weight-for-weight basis (Goodman and Gilman, 1975); pharmacokinetic data are not available. The phenomenon of the 'failed Palfium' patient is, however, only too familiar to those working with terminal cancer patients. Typically, such a patient has very severe or overwhelming pain and is taking 5–10 mg (1–2 tablets) every hour, or 15–20 mg every 2 hours. Partial or even complete relief is obtained for about $1-1\frac{1}{2}$ hours and for this reason the patient continues to take it. In short, dextromoramide would appear to be a potent but relatively short-lasting analgesic. Not infrequently this results in a vicious 'switchback' effect which increases the likelihood of the pain becoming even more severe. As a general rule, dextromoramide should be used only as a required second potent analgesic. If used on its own regularly, its use must be closely monitored, particularly in relation to duration of effect.

Initial dose of diamorphine

Sooner or later most doctors transfer their patients to diamorphine or morphine. Care must be taken to avoid, as far as possible, initiating treatment with an inadequate dose. An elderly patient prescribed diamorphine for generalized discomfort will usually be much helped by 2·5 mg 4-hourly. The same dose may be adequate when transferring from aspirin or paracetamol, though 5–10 mg will generally be necessary if converting from a weak narcotic. If, however, the patient has been receiving phenazocine, a much higher dose will be required (Fig. 5.5).

Because their pain has been eased fairly well for short periods, patients who have been taking 5–10 mg of dextromoramide every 1 or 2 hours are often reluctant to stop it until it has been demonstrated that the alternative offered is more efficacious. As a result, they may need to remain on dextromoramide initially until their confidence has been gained. One might prescribe, for example, diamorphine 20 mg plus dextromoramide 10 mg 4-hourly, converting to diamorphine 40–60 mg a few days later. Changing from methadone is more difficult as there will be a considerable 'carry-over' effect. If the methadone has been given 8- or 6-hourly, it would not be unreasonable to give double the dose of diamorphine 4-hourly. This may, however, be inadequate. In these circumstances, it is necessary to monitor the dose carefully for at least 3–4 days to prevent either break-through pain or over-sedation.

Adjuvant medication

Most patients with advanced cancer have more than one symptom, often

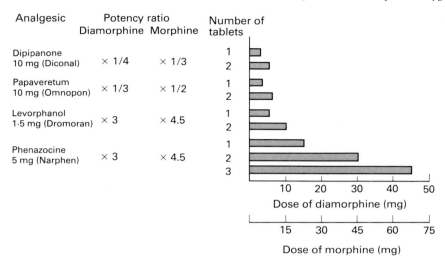

Fig. 5.5. Chart of approximate analgesic equivalence to oral diamorphine and morphine.

necessitating the prescription of several drugs at the same time. Moreover, use of narcotic analgesics is frequently complicated by constipation and/or nausea and vomiting. Any discussion of analgesics in advanced cancer must therefore include adjuvant medication.

Amiphenazole

It has been claimed that the use of amiphenazole (Daptazole), a respiratory stimulant, permits more rapid adjustment of morphine dosage as it antagonizes the respiratory depressant effect of the opiate (Shaw and Shulman, 1955). However, in a controlled trial of morphine with and without amiphenazole, it was demonstrated in non-tolerant, ex-addict volunteers that the addition of amiphenazole (1·2 mg for each mg of morphine) had no demonstrable effect on respiratory rate or volume. Injections of up to 120 mg of morphine were used four times a day (Fraser, Isbell and Van Horn, 1957).

In fact, significant respiratory depression is rarely a problem when opiates are used by mouth in individually determined doses. Patients with tachypnoea, often feel considerably better if, for example, the respiratory rate is reduced from 40 to 25 a minute. With this observation in mind, one should consider raising the dose of diamorphine or morphine, even if pain is controlled, in order to ease dyspnoea. In patients with a normal respiratory rate, it is unusual for this to fall below about 12 a minute. Individuals most at risk include the elderly, those receiving opiates by injection, and those who require an above-average dose of diamorphine or morphine together with diazepam or methotrimeprazine (see below). In these patients the rate may drop as low as 4–6 when the patient is asleep, a fact which naturally concerns the nurses. Occasionally, in an elderly patient, the medication may need to be modified if poor oxygenation precipitates or aggravates confusion; the need to do this is, however, uncommon.

Cocaine

More than 80 years ago, Herbert Snow (1896) began to prescribe cocaine with opium or morphine for patients with advanced cancer. He maintained that cocaine helped to 'sustain vitality', though subsequently he had to stop using it because of the cost. Thirty years later it was re-introduced by J. E. H. Roberts, a surgeon at the Brompton Hospital, who used a morphine–cocaine elixir as a post-thoracotomy analgesic (Kerrane, 1975). The mixture subsequently became known as the Brompton Cocktail. Since 1973, the British Pharmaceutical Codex has included a standard formulation for both morphine–cocaine and diamorphine–cocaine elixirs.

The addition of cocaine is said to enhance the mood of the patient; 'The euphoria renders the patient comparatively cheerful, and relieves his mental and physical distress' (Love, 1962). Only recently, however, has the effect of a standard 10 mg dose of cocaine hydrochloride been evaluated (Twycross, 1976). In this study patients were stabilized on morphine–cocaine, or diamorphine–cocaine, or morphine alone or diamorphine alone. After 2 weeks, patients receiving cocaine stopped receiving it, and vice versa. Stopping cocaine appeared to have no effect, though starting it resulted in a small but definite improvement in feelings of alertness and strength. This observation suggested that, when cocaine is given in a small fixed dose, tolerance develops after a few days. Cocaine would thus be of benefit during the initiation of treatment with morphine or diamorphine, but thereafter would be relatively ineffective.

Many physicians have, however, had experience of patients—usually elderly—who have become restless, agitated, confused and/or hallucinated when prescribed an opiate–cocaine mixture and whose symptoms have persisted until the cocaine was withdrawn. In view of this, and the equivocal nature of the trial results, the author no longer prescribes cocaine concomitantly. Instead, the patient is told that he may feel drowsy for 2 or 3 days following the start of treatment, but subsequently the drowsiness will become less. If the drowsiness persists, dexamphetamine 5 mg or methylphenidate (Ritalin) 10 mg may be prescribed once or twice daily.

Phenothiazines

Patients prescribed a narcotic analgesic should be questioned about nausea and vomiting and either have an antiemetic such as prochlorperazine prescribed simultaneously, or the need for such reviewed after 1 or 2 days. A patient will not continue to take an analgesic if it results in nausea or vomiting (see Chapter 6). In patients with an appreciable psychological component to their pain—for example, the patient with lung cancer experiencing both pain and dyspnoea and who fears death by suffocation, or the woman who feels that her fungating breast cancer is jeopardizing her relationship with her husband —promazine or chlorpromazine should be used instead. If the latter causes troublesome anticholinergic side-effects, it may be necessary to use prochlorperazine with diazepam; in the absence of nausea and vomiting the latter can, of course, be used alone. Promazine and chlorpromazine are also used to control confusion, delirium, or psychotic manifestations.

Whereas promazine and chlorpromazine merely potentiate the analgesic effect of narcotics, methotrimeprazine (Nozinan) possesses analgesic properties *per se* (Lasagna, 1965). By injection, methotrimeprazine 15 mg and morphine 10 mg are equipotent (Bonica and Halpern, 1972). The oral potency ratio has not been determined, but when allowance is made for differences between absorption and plasma half-time, it is possible that methotrimeprazine is at least as potent as morphine on a weight-for-weight basis. Its use in terminal pain is, however, limited because it is too sedative for most patients, causing unacceptable drowsiness. Methotrimeprazine also commonly causes marked orthostatic hypotension; because of this effect, some would restrict its use to non-ambulant patients. However, provided one is aware of the problem, this is unnecessary. Its use should be considered in the younger, anxious patient, requiring above average amounts of a narcotic and in those who experience marked vestibular disturbances when given a morphine-like drug. In those aged under 40, it would be reasonable to prescribe 25 mg 4- to 6-hourly with 50–100 mg at night; in older patients, the dose should be reduced by 50 per cent. As a rule of thumb, *the dose of morphine or diamorphine should be halved when prescribing methotrimeprazine for the first time.*

Benzodiazepines

Many patients appear to be psychologically dependent on nitrazepam as a night hypnotic and it may be necessary to continue this 'for old times' sake'. Diazepam is a useful alternative to promazine or chlorpromazine if side-effects make their use less attractive or if response is inadequate. It is also useful as a co-analgesic in muscle spasm pain and for urethral pain associated with an indwelling catheter.

Antidepressants

The need for an antidepressant increases the longer a patient is maintained on a narcotic analgesic (Twycross and Wald, 1976). Whether the onset of depression is precipitated by the protracted terminal illness itself or is a side-effect of long-continued treatment with a narcotic and a phenothiazine is not clear. It is important to be aware that depression not only can, but frequently does, supervene in patients receiving so-called 'euphoriant' drugs, and to initiate a trial of therapy when it does. Treatment should be started with half the usual adult dose, as experience has shown that debilitated patients commonly become confused and disorientated if a higher dose is given initially, particularly if they are receiving other psychotropic drugs.

As might be expected, not all patients respond to an antidepressant. If after a reasonable trial of therapy no effect is noted, treatment should be stopped. In these circumstances, alternative measures to be considered include:

1. Use of corticosteroids, e.g. prednisolone.
2. Prescription of amphetamine.
3. Change of environment, e.g. temporary admission to an hospice or similar unit.

Support and companionship are always necessary, particularly in cases where the depression is more properly described as sadness at the thought of leaving behind one's family, friends and all that is familiar.

Anti-inflammatory drugs

The use of these is described below in relation to bone and nerve compression pains.

Laxatives

Constipation almost always occurs and requires an appropriate regimen of diet, laxatives, suppositories and/or enemas (see Chapter 6).

Addiction

Although the term 'drug addiction' has been replaced officially by 'drug dependence', unofficially it continues to be used. Drug dependence is currently defined as:

'A state, psychic and sometimes also physical, resulting from the interaction between a living organism and a drug, characterized by behavioural and other responses that always include a compulsion to take the drug on a continuous or periodic basis in order to experience its psychic effects, and sometimes to avoid the discomfort of its absence. Tolerance may or may not be present' (World Health Organization, 1969).

This is a broader definition than an earlier one which emphasized the need for both tolerance and an early development of physical dependence in addition to strong psychological dependence (World Health Organization, 1964). The term 'drug dependence' now more closely approximates to the popular conception of addiction—a compulsion or overpowering drive to take the drug in order to experience its psychological effects. Occasionally a patient is admitted who appears to be addicted, demanding 'an injection' every 2 or 3 hours. Typically such a patient has a long history of poor pain control and will for several weeks have been receiving fairly regular ('four-hourly as required') but inadequate injections of one or more narcotic analgesics. Given time, it is usually possible to control the pain adequately, prevent clock-watching and demanding behaviour, and, sometimes, transfer the patient on to an oral preparation. But even here, it cannot be said that the patient is addicted as he is not demanding the narcotic in order to experience its psychological effect but to be relieved from pain for at least an hour or two.

Even so, many doctors are reluctant to use narcotic analgesics, particularly diamorphine or morphine, because they assume that tolerance will result in the medication becoming ineffective (Milton, 1972). This is understandable, as hitherto little information has been available concerning the long-term effects of narcotic analgesics when administered regularly to relieve persistent pain. The lack of data resulted in predictions being made on the basis of animal and human volunteer studies. For example, in a review article on narcotic analgesics (Martin, 1973), comments about tolerance in patients were supported by references, on the one hand, to a short-term infusion study in pain-free dogs and, on the other, to ex-addicts. However, in studies using ex-addicts at the Addiction Research Centre in Lexington, the emphasis has been on inducing tolerance and physical dependence as rapidly as possible by using maximum tolerated doses rather than administering the drugs in doses and at intervals comparable to a clinical regimen (Isbell, 1948). Although such studies have been useful in predicting abuse liability, their relevance to clinical practice is questionable.

To allow predictions to be made on the basis of clinical experience, the author has reviewed the notes of a considerable number of patients admitted to St Christopher's Hospice and who received diamorphine regularly to relieve pain associated with far-advanced cancer (Twycross, 1974b; Twycross and Wald, 1976). Initially, the notes of over 400 patients admitted consecutively were examined. Of median age 63 years, their median survival after admission was 16 days (range 1 day to 2 years). More than 60 per cent of these patients were maintained on a dose of 10 mg or less and only 8 per cent required more than a 30 mg dose. To examine the rate of increase in dose, patients were grouped according to survival, excluding the 213 who died within a week of commencing treatment. By plotting the median final daily dose for each group against the median duration of treatment it was demonstrated that *the longer the duration of treatment the slower the rate of rise in dose* (Fig. 5.6).

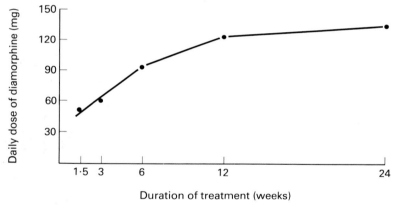

Fig. 5.6. 418 patients admitted consecutively with advanced cancer were grouped according to survival following the start of treatment with diamorphine; group median final daily dose of diamorphine is shown plotted against group median duration of treatment.

In a second review (Twycross and Wald, 1976), 115 patients who had received diamorphine regularly for at least 12 weeks were selected from approximately 3000 patients admitted over a period of years. Dose–time charts were prepared. Visual analysis indicated that in many there was an initial phase when the dose was increased several times followed by a prolonged phase when the dose was increased less often or not at all. The following definitions were applied:

Phase of initial pain control (phase 1)—from the beginning of treatment until the beginning of the first 'plateau' or 'plateau-descent'. A plateau was defined as any period of 2 weeks or more during which the dose of diamorphine was not increased, and a plateau-descent as any period of 2 weeks or more during which the dose of diamorphine was reduced.

Phase of continuing pain control (phase 2)—from the beginning of the first plateau-descent.

Phase of terminal pain control (phase 3)—from the end of the last plateau or plateau-descent until death.

Phase 1 was present on more than two-thirds of the dose–time charts. The mean length, including all 115 patients, was 8 days (SD ± 8) with an average rate of rise of 6 mg per day. Phase 3 was recorded in 64 patients, and its mean length was 5 days (SD ± 7) with an average rate of rise of 18 mg per day although in 48 of these, this simply reflected one or two dose adjustments within 2 weeks of death. The one constant feature of all 115 dose–time charts was the phase of continuing pain control. On average, patients had three periods of more than 6 weeks when the dose either remained the same or was reduced; the overall rate of change during this phase was 0·64 mg per day. Patients were divided into five groups according to survival (Table 5.6). Not

Table 5.6   Numerical analysis of Phase 2

	Group 1	Group 2	Group 3	Group 4	Group 5	Total
Survival (weeks)	12–13	14–17	18–25	26–41	42+	
Number	23	22	32	19	19	115
Average rate of change (mg/day)	+0·46	+1·45	+1·02	+0·29	+0·02	+0·64
Direction of dose change:						
Up	17	19	24	11	11	82
Down	4	2	5	6	7	24
No overall change	2	1	3	2	1	9
Number of plateaux	35	36	48	31	48	198
Number of plateau-descents	14	17	41	25	48	145
Average number of plateaux per patient	2	2·5	3	3	5	3
Average duration (days)	33	30	43	66	51	45

After Twycross and Wald (1976)

only did the average number of plateaux and plateau-descents increase from group 1 to 5, but their average duration increased from approximately 4 to 8 weeks. (The apparent 'fall-off' in group 5 is because one patient who is still alive after 5 years required diamorphine for only 16 weeks.) Further, there was a definite increase in the ratio of plateau-descents to plateaux as one moved from group 1 to group 5 ($p < 0·01$). *This means that the longer a patient survived after prescription of diamorphine, the greater the likelihood of a reduction in dose.*

Dose reductions were made on a trial and error basis in patients who had improved generally over a number of weeks and who had had no recent episodes of 'breakthrough' pain. Reductions were also made after successful intrathecal nerve blocks in 5 patients and after treatment with a cytotoxic agent or radiation in a number of others. A total of 9 patients, all in group 5, stopped receiving diamorphine: 3 stopped taking diamorphine altogether; 4 patients stopped for more than 4 months; and 2 stopped for approximately 3 weeks.

It was concluded that, when used as part of a pattern of total care, diamorphine may be used for long periods without concern about tolerance. Moreover, although physical dependence probably develops in most patients after several weeks of continuous treatment (Eddy, Lee and Harris, 1959), this does not prevent the downward adjustment of dose when considered clinically feasible. Experience with methadone (Nathan, 1952), levorphanol and phenazocine suggests that the 'natural history' of their long-term use for patients in pain is similar to that of diamorphine and morphine.

Case histories

The following case histories, all of women with breast cancer, highlight many of the points discussed in this chapter.

1. Mrs V.N. (54)

A year after mastectomy she developed anorexia with nausea and vomiting. She lost weight, became progressively weaker and, finally, bedfast. In addition, she had severe pain in the lumbar spine which radiated down the back of the right leg. On admission her prognosis was estimated to be less than 1 week; she was prescribed diamorphine and promazine. Within a few days she was able to sit in a chair for short periods. She developed pain in the cervical spine and it was necessary to increase the dose of diamorphine on two occasions (Fig. 5.7a). After 4 weeks, prednisone 20 mg/24 h was prescribed and a few days later the previously persistent nausea diminished and her appetite increased. She continued to improve and was fully mobile after 2 months. The diamorphine was reduced and the patient subsequently discharged. She was readmitted after 2 weeks, anxious and depressed, but improved following the prescription of imipramine. She went home on several occasions for the day and was discharged again after 2 months. Eight months later she was admitted for a course of chemotherapy following recurrence of back pain which radiated down both legs. Her final admission was precipitated by depression which was helped by increasing the dose of imipramine. Five weeks later the back pain recurred and she complained of numbness in the feet and absence of urethral sensation. For the last 5 weeks it was necessary to administer diamorphine by injection in order to relieve the pain. She died 2 years after her first admission.

Comment

The patient was almost certainly hypercalcaemic when admitted, and improved rapidly and dramatically when prednisone was prescribed. Hypercalcaemia is known to precipitate or exacerbate pain in breast cancer and its correction to cause relief (Galasko and Burn, 1971). Several of the upward adjustments in the dose of diamorphine were for pain associated with different metastatic lesions. Other adjustments related to a lesion in the lumbar spine which, as it progressed, caused first unilateral sciatic pain, then bilateral sciatic pain and, finally, symptoms suggestive of spinal cord compression. At one point, chemotherapy was used in addition to the diamorphine and other medication. Despite receiving diamorphine with cocaine and prednisone, the patient became depressed and required an antidepressant. Three of the six admissions were precipitated by anxiety and/or depression.

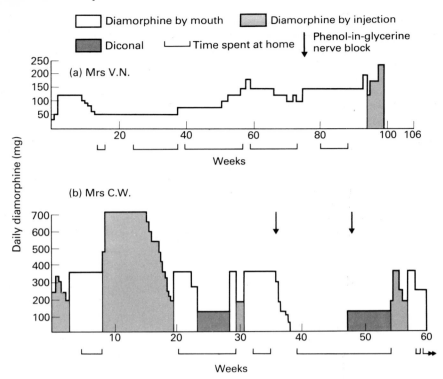

Fig. 5.7. Dose–time charts of (a) Mrs V.N. (case history 1) and (b) Mrs C.W. (case history 2).

2. Mrs C.W. (33)

The mother of two young children had cancer of the left breast, diagnosed 4 years before. This was treated by mastectomy and radiotherapy. She subsequently had an oophorectomy and, a year later, a hypophysectomy. The patient spent most of the day lying flat in bed on account of severe pain caused by a metastasis in the lumbar spine. She also complained of intermittent nausea and retching and was breathless on exertion. When admitted, she was receiving oral diamorphine and dipipanone with cyclizine (Diconal) four-hourly. Parenteral diamorphine, oral chlorpromazine and phenylbutazone were prescribed (Fig. 5.7b).

The patient was mobilized increasingly once the pain was relieved and was discharged on oral medication after 5 weeks. X-rays showed partial collapse of L4. She was subsequently readmitted several times because of exacerbations of lower back pain. The diamorphine was tailed off after an intrathecal nerve block but she continued to take phenylbutazone and dextropropoxyphene plus paracetamol (Distalgesic). A second block was not as successful and Diconal was necessary to control the pain. She was later prescribed diamorphine and chlorpromazine. Both the patient and family required continued support. Diazepam was prescribed at times of additional stress and trimipramine (used as night sedative) was replaced by amitriptyline after 14 months. The patient died 2 years after her first admission.

Comment

The patient required a large parenteral dose of diamorphine for exacerbation of pain but, each time, was subsequently able to revert to oral medication. On two occasions diamorphine was stopped altogether at the patient's request: (1) when she was transferred to an alternative preparation (Diconal), and (2) after the first nerve block. Both the patient and her family needed considerable, continuing support.

3. Mrs V.H. (62)

This patient developed skeletal metastases 5 years after mastectomy for carcinoma of the left breast. She sustained a pathological fracture of the neck of left femur which was pinned and plated. When admitted, she complained of pain in the left hip and walked with crutches. She was initially prescribed dihydrocodeine and cyclizine. Exacerbation of the pain a week later resulted in the prescription of diamorphine, chlorpromazine and prednisone. She became fully mobile but subsequently experienced episodes of renewed pain which related to fresh metastatic activity. The dose of diamorphine was increased when necessary. Eventually she was able to go home but, after 3 months, was readmitted with pneumonia and died after a few hours.

Comment

The dose–time chart shows three elevations (Fig. 5.8a). The first and third relate to a new pain caused by fresh metastactic activity. In the second elevation, the recurrence of a previous pain led to the increase. At first sight, then, tolerance to diamorphine might be suspected. However, the ability to make a fourfold reduction in dose some 3 weeks later suggests that this elevation also resulted from an acute episode relating to a skeletal metastasis. The final

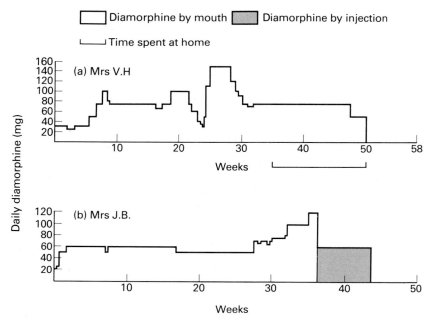

Fig. 5.8. Dose–time charts of (a) Mrs V.H. (case history 3) and (b) Mrs J.B. (case history 4).

reduction, made by the patient's general practitioner, led to recurrence of intermittent discomfort, demonstrating that the patient still required analgesics at this stage.

4. Mrs J.B. (45)

This patient had been treated by irradiation for disseminated bilateral breast cancer nine months before admission. This had been followed by radiotherapy to the left breast and lumbar spine. When admitted, she was paraplegic and complained of nausea and vomiting. There was a large mass in the hypogastrium which, when moved, caused severe pain to shoot down both legs. She was frightened and tearful and, when asked why she had let her breasts get so bad, she replied because she was afraid it was something awful. Diamorphine and chlorpromazine were prescribed (Fig. 5.8b). After 4 weeks amitriptyline was added. She gradually became less tearful. There were, however, considerable family problems and her mood remained variable. A pathological fracture of the right femur was treated conservatively. Latterly, she was drowsy for most of the time and slept for long periods. After 9 months she was transferred to parenteral therapy, and died peacefully of pneumonia 7 weeks later.

Comment

The patient and her family needed considerable support during the illness. Because of paraplegia she remained in hospital throughout the terminal stage of her illness. It is not possible to say whether the drowsiness related to treatment or to the underlying disease. There are, however, occasions when some impairment of consciousness must be accepted as the price of adequate relief. The degree of drowsiness was not, however, constant; Mrs J.B. was able to enjoy her visitors and, to within a few weeks of death, she was alert and talkative for some part of most days.

Bone pain

Metastases in bone are a common cause of pain in disseminated malignant disease, especially in carcinomas of the breast, bronchus and prostate. As bone pain is not always relieved by analgesics alone, it may be necessary to use several measures simultaneously to obtain relief. These include measures which modify tumour growth (radiation, chemotherapy, endocrine manipulation) and chemical neurolysis (see the Addendum to this chapter).

As the cancer progresses, however, and attempts to palliate the disease become less effective, the use of analgesics and other measures to elevate the pain threshold become increasingly important. Clinical experience suggests that the combined use of both a narcotic and a potent anti-inflammatory analgesic, such as phenylbutazone, indomethacin or aspirin, yields better results than use of the former alone. Phenylbutazone, up to 200 mg 4-hourly, is perhaps the best tolerated of the three. Although not a steroid, phenylbutazone causes a variable degree of sodium and water retention. Gastrointestinal symptoms may occur with all three drugs, especially with indomethacin. The usual dose of indomethacin is 25 mg four times a day which, as far as possible, should be taken after meals. If aspirin is used, a daily dose of at least 3·4 g is required to achieve a definite anti-inflammatory effect.

Alternatively, prednisolone 5–10 mg three times a day may be used. This has a number of added advantages; it elevates mood and stimulates appetite (Moertel *et al.*, 1974; Twycross, in preparation), and often corrects associated hypercalcaemia (Watson, 1972), though gastric irritation and fluid retention may occur.

Recent work has clarified the basis for the use of non-steroidal anti-inflammatory drugs in the relief of bone pain. Certain prostaglandins, particularly of the E series, induce osteolysis and can also cause pain at high concentrations, probably by sensitizing nerve endings. Aspirin and other non-steroidal anti-inflammatory drugs are known to be potent inhibitors of prostaglandin synthetase. It seems, therefore, that these drugs not only relieve pain by reducing the local concentration of PGE_2 but also impede the continued growth of metastases in bone.

Response to prostaglandin inhibitors is, however, variable, and it is likely that several other pharmacological and enzymatic factors may mediate bone destruction. As further research elucidates the relative importance of these substances, the ability to relieve bone pain by pharmacological means should steadily improve.

Pathological fracture

Internal fixation or the insertion of a prosthesis should be considered if a pathological fracture of a long bone occurs; such measures obviate the need for prolonged bedrest and pain is usually much reduced. The decision whether to treat surgically depends on the patient's general condition; however, whereas in bronchial carcinoma pathological fracture often presages death, in breast cancer this is not generally so. In 13 breast cancer patients whose illness was complicated by pathological fracture, either before or after admission to St Christopher's Hospice, median survival following the first or only fracture was 5 months, ranging from 2 months to 4 years.

Recently, it has been suggested that when pathological fracture is likely the long bone should be nailed prophylactically, as this is simpler than the internal fixation of an established displaced fracture, and less disturbing for the patient. Prophylactic nailing facilitates nursing and usually results in considerable reduction of pain. Moreover, even when a fracture occurs after nailing it can be virtually symptomless. Parrish and Murray (1970) described 4 cases where the indication for prophylactic internal fixation was increasing pain combined with destruction of more than 50 per cent of the cortex. When more than half of the cortex has been destroyed, deformity takes place on weight-bearing and causes pain in a similar manner to a stress fracture; this is prevented by internal fixation.

Fidler (1973) reviewed 19 fractures through metastases, 18 in the femur. He confirmed that fracture was unlikely when less than 25 per cent of the cortex had been eroded but that with over 75 per cent involvement the bone was so weak as often to fracture spontaneously. Further, he emphasized that, although pain may draw attention to a metastasis, it was not helpful in deciding whether a fracture was likely. In fact only half his patients had pain before the fracture. He concluded that destruction of 50 per cent of the cortex was indication for prophylactic internal fixation, and cited 9 operations. In 1, the femur fractured during surgery, but in none did a pathological fracture follow the operation.

A more elaborate technique has been described for use when bone destruction is widespread or when the fracture is close to the end of the bone and adequate fixation by a nail is not possible (Harrington *et al.*, 1972); lesions are first treated by excision and curettage and then by appropriate internal fixation and the simultaneous insertion of an acrylic cement into the bone defect. However, because of the possibility of tumour dissemination, routine curettage is probably not advisable. The selective use of acrylic cement without curettage will still allow the fixation of fractures which would otherwise not be manageable (Editorial, 1976).

Nerve compression pain

Analgesics are often effective in relieving pain due to nerve compression. If the response is poor, however, the use of prednisolone 5–10 mg three times a day is recommended. By reducing inflammatory swelling round the growth, the effective tumour mass is reduced and the compression alleviated. In patients with a prognosis of only a few weeks, this may be sufficient to circumvent the need for chemical neurolysis. In those with a longer life expectancy, the pain may return as the tumour continues to grow; in these a nerve block will be required. In patients whose morale is low or precarious, it may be advisable to warn that a block may become necessary, in order to avoid loss of confidence should the pain return. Equally, it is important that such patients should be reviewed regularly to prevent undue delay in the event of a resurgence of pain (see the Addendum to this chapter).

Other measures

When fungation occurs, and with oropharyngeal malignancies, some of the pain may be caused by inflammation secondary to infection. The concomitant use of an antibiotic will help considerably in these cases. Pain associated with lymphoedema of the arm is often helped by the regular use of a Flowtron or Jobst compression unit, whether or not the swelling is measurably decreased.

Headache due to raised intracranial pressure is best treated by a potent corticosteroid such as dexamethasone 2–4 mg three times a day and an analgesic. If diamorphine or morphine become necessary, the dose may have to be increased progressively as the resultant elevation in $PaCO_2$ will cause a further rise in intracranial pressure which will tend to make the headache worse.

Diversional therapy is also important. This includes backrubs, talking books, access to radio and television, someone to talk to, craft work and dayroom activities. Pain feels worse when it occupies the patient's whole attention. Diversional activity does more than just 'pass the time': it also diminishes the pain. In short, there is much more to analgesia than analgesics. This means that success will be achieved more readily if the problem is tackled in a comprehensive manner.

'I would suggest that the successful therapist for intractable pain treats the problem like a game in which he endeavours to outmanoeuvre the tricks performed by the central nervous system of his patient. He has many different moves he can play. Some depend on simple procedures which checkmate the mechanisms, but others are assisted by the deception of the poker player and the confidence of the quack' (Russell. 1959).

References

AITKEN-SWAN, J. (1959). *Practitioner* **183**, 64.

BONICA, J. J. and HALPERN, L. M. (1972). Analgesics. In: *Drugs of Choice, 1972–1973*. Ed. by W. Modell. Mosby; St. Louis.

DUBOISSON, D. and MELZACK, R. (1976). *Experimental Neurology* **51**, 480.

DUNDEE, J. W. and JONES, P. O. (1968). *British Journal of Clinical Practice* **22**, 379.

EDDY, N. B., LEE, L. E. and HARRIS, C. A. (1959). *Bulletin on Narcotics* **11**, 1, 3.

EDITORIAL (1976). *Lancet* **2**, 943.

FIDLER, M. (1973). *British Medical Journal* **1**, 341.

FRASER, H. F., ISBELL, H. and VAN HORN, G. D. (1957). *Anesthiology* **18**, 531.

GALASKO, C. S. B. and BURN, J. I. (1971). *British Medical Journal* **3**, 573.

GLYNN, C. J., LLOYD, J. W. and FOLKARD, S. (1976). *Proceedings of the Royal Society of Medicine* **69**, 369.

GOODMAN, L. S. and GILMAN, A, (1975). *The Pharmacological Basis of Therapeutics*, 5th ed. Macmillan, New York, London and Toronto.

HARRINGTON, K. D., JOHNSTON, J. O., TURNER, R. H. and GREEN, D. L. (1972). *Journal of Bone and Joint Surgery* **54A**, 1665.

HOUDE, R. W., WALLENSTEIN, S. L. and BEAVER, W. T. (1965). Clinical measurement of pain. In: *Analgetics*. Ed. by G. de Stevens. Academic Press; New York and London.

HUNT, J. M., STOLLAR, T. D., LITTLEJOHNS, D. W., TWYCROSS, R. G. and VERE, D. W. (1977). *Journal of Medical Ethics* **3**, 61.

ISBELL (1948). *Annals of New York Academy of Science* **51**, 108.

KERRANE, T. A. (1973). *Nursing Mirror* **140**, 59.

LASAGNA (1965). *Proceedings of the Royal Society of Medicine* **58**, 978.

LOVE, M. (1962). *British Medical Journal* **2**, 1192.

MARKS, R. H. and SACHAR, E. J. (1973). *Annals of International Medicine* **78**, 173.

MARTIN, W. R. (1973). *British Journal of Hospital Medicine* **10**, 173.

MARTINDALE (1977). *Extra Pharmacopoeia*, 27th edn. Pharmaceutical Press; London.

MILLER, R. R., FEINGOLD, A. and PAXINOS, J. (1970). *Journal of the American Medical Association* **213**, 996.

MILTON, G. W. (1972). *Medical Journal of Australia* **2**, 177.

MOERTAL, C. G., SCHUTT, A. J., REITEMEIER, R. J. and HAHN, R. G. (1974). *Cancer* **33**, 1607.

NATHAN, P. W. (1952). *British Medical Journal* **2**, 903.

PARKES, C. M. (1977). Evaluation of family care in terminal illness. In: *The Family and Death*. Ed. by E. R. Pritchard, J. Collard, B. A. Orcutt, A. H. Kutscher, I. Seeland and N. Lefkowicz. Columbia University Press; New York.

PARRISH, F. F. and MURRAY, J. A. (1970). *Journal of Bone and Joint Surgery* **52A**, 665.

ROBBIE, D. S. and SAMARASINGHE, J. (1973). *Journal of International Medical Research* **1**, 246.

RUSSELL, W. R. (1959). *Proceedings of the Royal Society of Medicine* **52**, 983.

SEED, J. C., WALLENSTEIN, S. L., HOUDE, R. W. and BELVILLE, J. W. (1958). *Archives Internationales de Pharmacodynamie et de Therapie* **116**, 293.

SHAW, F. H. and SHULMAN, A. (1955). *British Medical Journal* **1**, 1367.

SMITHERS, D. (1973). *British Medical Journal* **1**, 34.

SNOW, H. (1896). *British Medical Journal* **2**, 718.

TURNBULL, F. (1954). *Proceedings of the Royal Society of Medicine* **47**, 155.

TWYCROSS, R. G. (1974a). *Pharmaceutical Journal* **212**, 153, 159.

TWYCROSS, R. G. (1974b). *International Journal of Clinical Pharmacology, Therapy and Toxicology* **9**, 184.

TWYCROSS, R. G. (1976). *Studies on the use of diamorphine in advanced malignant disease*. DM Thesis (Oxford).

TWYCROSS, R. G. (1977). *Pain* **3**, 93.

TWYCROSS, R. G. and WALD, S. J. (1976). The long-term use of diamorphine in advanced cancer. In: *Advances in Pain Research and Therapy*, vol. 1, p. 653. Ed. by J. J. Bonica and D. Albe-Faescard. Raven Press; New York.

TWYCROSS, R. G., FRY, D. E. and WILLS, P. D. (1974). *British Journal of Clinical Pharmacology* **1**, 491.

VEREBELY, K., VOLAVKA, J., MULE, S. and RESNICK, R. (1975). *Clinical Pharmacology and Therapeutics* **18**, 180.

WATSON, L. (1972). *British Medical Journal* **2**, 150.

WAY, E. L., YOUNG, J. M. and KEMP, J. W. (1965). *Bulletin on Narcotics* **17**, No. 1., 25.

WOOD, A. J. J., NOIR, D. C., CAMPBELL, C., DAVIDSON, J. F., GALLON, S. E., HENNY, E. and McALLION, S. (1974). *British Medical Journal* **1**, 305.

World Health Organization (1964). *Expert Committee on Drug Dependence, 13th Report, Technical Report Series No. 287.*

World Health Organization (1969). *Expert Committee on Drug Dependence, 16th Report, Technical Report Series No. 407.*

Addendum
Nerve Blocks and Other Procedures

D. S. Robbie

In certain circumstances it is both desirable and feasible to relieve the pain of terminal cancer by special procedures such as nerve blocks. This short account will deal with certain nerve block techniques which can be carried out in situations without a full general hospital facility, including the patient's own home.

Pain sensations are carried in the smallest nerve fibres and these are damaged by neurolytic agents more completely and in greater numbers than larger nerve fibres which mediate other sensory stimuli and motor power. This selective pattern of fibre damage is the expected outcome when a peripheral mixed nerve is blocked at any point extending from the extradural areas outside the coverings of the spinal cord (dura arachnoid) to the point of innervation. The area where the patient feels pain may be distant from the irritant lesion. Sciatic pain, for example, may be associated with pelvic cancer, and pain in the arm with neoplasms affecting the nerves in the neck. It is usually necessary to place the neurolytic solutions proximal to the lesion—which may be recurrent or metastatic cancer, local fibrosis following surgery or radiotherapy, or altered tissue reactions following cytotoxic drugs.

Intrathecal nerve blocking

The site of the lesion causing the pain may be so near the spinal cord that the introduction of neurolytic solutions into the dura arachnoid may have to be considered. This intrathecal area is approached by a spinal tap with a needle inserted between the laminae of the vertebrae, and a neurolytic solution deposited. The easiest and safest approach is by lumbar puncture, and many blocks can be attempted by this route. Solutions of phenol in glycerine are heavier than cerebrospinal fluid and are reliable in their effects. Solutions of from 5 to 7·5 per cent phenol are used in amounts of about 1 ml. The patient is positioned on his painful side for the lumbar puncture and, either before or after the installation of the heavy neurolytic solution, he is tilted backwards so that the injected solution is concentrated in the posterior part of the cerebro-spinal space where the sensory nerve roots lie (rather than in the anterior part where the motor nerve roots emerge). The patient remains in position for 30–60 minutes to allow the phenol to be completely absorbed onto the appropriate posterior sensory roots and nerve ganglia.

Initially, intrathecal nerve blocks are carried out on an operating theatre table with the patient fully conscious and able to advise the operator of areas of numbness or motor paralysis as and when they occur. The patient is positioned by altering the shape and tilts of the operating table. The technique is a 'blind' one and, initially, it is rarely possible to be certain of affecting the sensory nerve roots in a completely selective fashion. There must be a tendency for the glycerine vehicle to settle in the intervertebral foramina where the motor and sensory roots meet. There may therefore be local paralysis immediately after a block, which passes off within 30 minutes; on the other hand, numbness—and pain relief—continue. How long they continue depends on the individual. With experience and analysis of results, gross percentages can provide a reasonable guide to the good effects and undesirable effects of neurolytic techniques; however, individual response cannot be confidently predicted, and a cautious and conservative approach is prudent. In a personal series of 42 patients who had lumbosacral pain from pelvic cancer, 96 intrathecal nerve blocks were carried out with 5–7·5 per cent phenol in glycerine. Two patients had serious side-effects in the form of bladder paralysis and lower limb paresis; 19 patients had lesser side-effects such as increased bladder sphincter deficit up to 1 week, or numbness, paraesthesia or proprioceptive loss.

To begin with, a spinal block using local anaesthetic agents is carried out to assess the relief of pain obtained and the reaction of the patient to side-effects, including numbness. Nerve blocks with weak (5 per cent) phenol solutions are then carried out and repeated as indicated with stronger solutions of phenol, perhaps injected in greater quantity.

It is unnecessary to move a conscious patient with painful terminal cancer onto an operating table for a nerve block. It is possible to tip the patient's bed and use pillows to posture satisfactorily. It is, however, often difficult for the patient to lie on the painful side for the initial lumbar puncture and to hold this position comfortably—even if the block relieves severe pain at once. Many patients have a horror of lumbar puncture and additional sedation may be required, varying from added analgesics to intravenous diazepam to brief anaesthesia followed by sedation. This will limit the amount of communication with the patient!

The site where intrathecal blocks are most applicable is, however, the lum-bosacral area where problems of posturing are least taxing for the patient. The usual intention is to damage the lumbosacral sensory roots on one side, and a straightforward head-up tilt will be required with the patient tilted to the painful side lying on some pillows. As this position has to be maintained for up to 1 hour, intravenous diazepam is a useful sedative. Bilateral lumbosacral nerve blocks may be necessary if pain is central or bilateral.

The general problems of unwanted sensory loss and motor paresis associated with a neurolytic block have already been noted. These side-effects can become more objectionable to the patient the greater the relief of pain produced and the less sleepy he is from revised and reduced drug regimens. A particularly contentious issue is the loss of full bladder control after a neurolytic block in the lumbosacral region. This may be temporary, but about 25 per cent of patients will need an indwelling catheter for a period. Bladder control is often impaired in patients with pelvic cancer, and it may easily be lost with any further insult. I find that most patients who have this prospect put to them are reluctant to contemplate a nerve block, even with the prospect of relieving their pain; such response is reinforced when their terminal care is being well handled in hospital or home. (There is no such difficulty, of course, if the patient already has loss of bladder control or has an artificial bladder.)

A similar but lesser problem arises in relation to rectal control. Again, there is no difficulty if this has already been lost, or there is a functioning abdominal colostomy or ileostomy. Many patients are very constipated and any alteration of anorectal control passes almost unnoticed. A different situation occurs where the patient is dependent on good control for loose bowel motions.

Other sensory deficits usually accompany relief of pain. Most of these are disliked, whether they are experienced as pins and needles, numbness, or other forms of altered sensation; but the hope is that a more normal sensory state will return with few painful stimuli.

Loss of proprioceptive sensation adds to any motor paresis in causing ambulatory difficulties. Both usually return over the course of days or weeks, but the patient may feel seriously handicapped.

Intrathecal blocks may be used to relieve severe bladder spasm by damaging the innervation of the bladder through the sacral nerve roots. One first blocks the side which seems to be associated with the most disease, then repeats on the same side or the other side as symptoms and side-effects indicate.

Patients may have spastic paraplegia as a result of primary or metastatic tumour invading the spine and cord. The motor roots can be damaged by larger amounts of stronger phenol solutions (e.g. 10 ml of 10 per cent) allowing easier bed-nursing of the patient; sitting out of bed could be feasible. Such patients may also have very severe painful spasms added to their spastic paraplegia and these should be relieved as well. Other sensory and motor deficits are not usually of concern, as these unfortunate patients already have sensory loss, indwelling catheters and require manual removal of faeces.

Patients in pain who have had neurosurgery to the spinal cord for cancer often have abnormal loculations in the intrathecal space due to adhesions. A trial spinal block with local anaesthetic agents usually produces bizarre areas of anaesthesia because of the loculations; intrathecal neurolytic agents should not be used to relieve their pain.

Neurolytic agents can be placed in any part of the spinal canal and the general rules indicated for the lumbosacral areas must be considered relative to the different areas. The beginner would be wise to feel confident regarding the problems at the lower end of the spinal cord before venturing higher. Spinal tap is more difficult outside the lumbar area and there is a risk of damaging the cord itself if there is doubt about needle position. A brisk flow of cerebrospinal fluid is the main safeguard against actual injection of the cord with a potentially disastrous outcome. There is a natural curve in the mid-thoracic vertebral column and this tends to prevent glycerine solutions from going higher if injected below and lower if injected above that level.

Peripheral nerve blocking

Examples of blocks at three sites are briefly described; two of them—the brachial plexus and intercostal nerves—are made up of mixed somatic fibres, while the third—the coeliac plexus—is made up of autonomic fibres.

Brachial plexus nerve block

The peripheral nerves to and from the upper limb are gathered together in the supraclavicular fossa around the subclavian vessels on the first rib, behind the clavicle. Techniques and risks of carrying out this block are described by Lee and Atkinson (1973). The painful upper limb is not uncommon in cancers involving the neck, lung and breast and can present a difficult problem. Usually the pain will be accompanied by wasting and loss of function of parts of the upper limb, especially the hand, as well as loss of sensation. This is distressing to the patient, and an assessment of relief from a local anaesthetic nerve block may be worth while. In theory and usually in practice it is necessary to inject the solutions proximal to the lesion to obtain relief from pain; but the exact local lesion is often unclear and palpation of the supra-clavicular fossa will vary from normal to a hard indurated mass, depending on the spread of tumour and the effects of local treatment such as radiotherapy.

The block is carried out with the patient fully conscious or sedated. The upper limb will vary from numb to paralysed with the strength of local anaes-thetic agent used in a trial block. An assessment can be made as to the amount of pain relief possible and the likely resentment of the patient to prolonged numbness and motor loss if a nerve-destroying agent is used. In general, it is hard for the patient to agree to loss of power and sensation from the upper limb unless the arm is quite useless. Also there is often the expectation, based on previous information from doctors, that the situation in the upper limb will improve. The 'blocker' may find it necessary to modify the patient's exag-gerated expectations and perhaps talk in terms of temporary blocks to relief pain while the limb recovers.

Occasionally, bizarre results can occur from injecting local anaesthetic into a mass in the supraclavicular fossa, and delayed relief of pain can follow after some hours and pass off again very slowly. Similar effects then occur with the neurolytic agent.

If the patient agrees to a more permanent nerve block the operator can proceed by using different strengths and amounts of the neurolytic agents. The commonest agent to damage peripheral nerves is alcohol in strengths from 25 to 100 per cent. This can be made stronger by adding phenol, depending on the effect desired. The injection of these alcohol agents is painful, so either the requisite area is first infiltrated with local anaesthetic or the patient may require brief light anaesthesia or sedation to tolerate the discomfort, which is initially intense but decreases over a few minutes. It is vital to avoid intra-arterial infection of the neurolytic agents or gangrene may result. With all these blocks repetition is possible, if acceptable, and good results lasting several weeks can be obtained.

The beginner should familiarize himself with the techniques of the block using local anaesthetic before employing neurolytic agents. Local anaesthetic blocks may give more effective relief from pain than analgesic drugs; but how much of this improvement is due to altering the vicious cycle of pain, or reception of the pain, or to psychotherapy is unclear. Many patients, however, are reasonably maintained on local anaesthetic blocks repeated at variable periods of days or weeks.

Intercostal nerve blocks

Intercostal nerve blocking is straightforward at many points and is worth considering when the painful area involves the chest wall, parietal pleura, abdominal wall, parietal peritoneum or the peripheral parts of the diaphragm. The technique is described by Lee and Atkinson (1973) and the procedure is easiest where the ribs are felt readily.

Several nerves on one or both sides may have to be blocked and this is carried out proximal to the area to be numbed. A trial block with local anaesthetic is usually indicated and, as with other nerve blocks, the benefit may outlast the time of action of the local anaesthetics.

If the relief of pain is satisfactory then neurolytic solutions of alcohol, with or without phenol, can be used. Again, the injection of these is painful, so the patient will require to be sedated or anaesthetized, or have a local block first at the site of the permanent block or proximal to it. If the alcohol solutions are injected intrapleurally in error there can be severe pleuritic pain which requires sedation and rest for a few hours. With correct placement of the alcohol a mild chemical pleuritis occurs which subsides over a few days; relief of painful symptoms may last weeks. The area affected by the block will be numb and occasionally there is weakness noticed in the abdominal wall muscles.

With obese patients it may be more straightforward to give them a light anaesthetic and use a neurolytic solution initially, as locating the ribs may be difficult and therefore uncomfortable.

Coeliac plexus blocks

The automatic nerves also carry sensation. Sometimes it is possible to relieve the pain associated with upper abdominal or retroperitoneal tumours by coeliac plexus block. The organs which may be numbed include the stomach, liver, gall-bladder and pancreas. The coeliac plexus lies in front of the first lumbar vertebra and can be approached fairly readily from the paravertebral region below the last rib, as described by Lee and Atkinson. Simple techniques are quite reasonable to use for the treatment of terminal cancer pain although more advanced techniques, requiring radiological control, have been developed. With retroperitoneal tumours it may be difficult to achieve spread of fluids to affect the plexus. Usually the block is first carried out with local anaesthetic to assess the benefit and then repeated with neurolytic solutions depending on the benefit obtained. Doses of 20 ml of 50 per cent alcohol might be considered initially. For the patient with terminal cancer it may be more expeditious to use an alcohol solution initially under sedation as the neurolytic injection is distressing. The main complication of the block is light-headedness on sitting or standing up, which results from an increased blood distribution to the gut—a postural hypotension. This settles after a few days and the level of pain may be dramatically lessened. A more acceptable side-effect is an increased activity of the bowel which is now functioning under lessened sympathetic nerve control.

Miscellaneous special techniques

There are a number of other techniques which can be considered by the enthusiast with little technical backing.

Hypnosis

Hypnosis has been used to relieve the pain of cancer both in individual and group situations. Sometimes the patient can be taught autohypnosis. It is said that most doctors can be effective hypnotists and most patients can be hypnotized to levels where relief is given to their painful symptoms. With successful individual hypnosis a situation of personal dependence on the hypnotist is likely to develop and the time factor then involved becomes unmanageable in practice, or will lead to the hypnotist being emotionally and physically exhausted.

Acupuncture

Acupuncture is a topical mode of therapy and there are a variety of views as to how effective it is on its own account, or whether there are elements of hypnotherapy plus peripheral nerve stimulation altering the perception of pain. In most situations the effectiveness of treatment is of short duration and problems pertaining to the ready availability of a competent acupuncturist arise very much as with the hypnotist situation.

Peripheral nerve stimulators

In recent years there have been a variety of new neurosurgical procedures developed to alter the appreciation of pain by the patient, using electrical stimuli to the sensory nerve tracts in the spinal cord. In the wake of these operations portable electrical stimulators have been developed where currents of variable pattern are applied to the skin near the painful areas. The best results occur when the relief of pain continues after the actual use of the nerve stimulator. The advantage of this technique is that it can be carried out with safety by the patient or non-medical personnel at home or hospital. It is too early to be clear how helpful these mini-stimulators will be in cancer pain, but they are obviously related to occupational therapy and psychotherapy with distraction which provide variable support to patients with minimal side-effects. At the worst, the patient dislikes the technique as unpleasant, or may have increased pain for a limited time after use of the stimulator.

Nitrous oxide/oxygen mixtures

Mixtures of 50 per cent nitrous oxide and 50 per cent oxygen are readily available for self-administration from gas cylinders with a pressure-reducing valve and breathing attachments similar to anaesthetic tubes and masks. They are used with minimal medical and nursing supervision but depend on a close-fitting face-mask and reasonable energy to open the demand valve on inspiration. In selected cases they can be useful to cope with short-lasting severe pains as the effect comes on fairly quickly and passes off quickly. They also can be of help with pain involved in cleaning and dressing raw areas or other short but painful nursing or medical procedures.

Reference and further reading

BONICA, J. J. (1974). *Advances in Neurology*, Vol. 4. Raven Press; New York.
HANNINGTON-KIFF, J. G. (1974). *Pain Relief*. Heinemann Medical; London.
HART, F. D. (1974). *The Treatment of Chronic Pain*. Medical and Technical Publishing; Lancaster.
LEE, J. A. and ATKINSON, R. S. (1973). *A Synopsis of Anaesthesia*, Wright; Bristol.
LIPTON, S. (1976). *Recent Advances in Anaesthesia and Analgesia*. Ed. by C. L. Hewer and R. S. Atkinson. Churchill Livingstone; Edinburgh and London.
MEHTA, M. (1973). *Intractable Pain*. Saunders; London.
SWORDLOW, M. (1974). *Relief of Intractable Pain*. Excerpta Medica; London.

6

Control of Other Symptoms

Mary J. Baines

'When you know why, you know how.'

'Feverishness is generally supposed to be a symptom of fever—in nine cases out of ten it is a symptom of bedding.'
  Nightingale, 1946

Advanced malignancy commonly affects many organs in the body, disturbs the biochemical balance and may, among other effects, be associated with ectopic hormone production (see Chapter 2). Terminal care must involve careful attention to the multitude of symptoms which a patient may therefore develop in his last few weeks or months of life. As in general medicine, it is important to diagnose the cause of each symptom and to base treatment on it. This diagnosis should be based on a careful history and clinical examination rather than on frequent or lengthy investigations (see Chapter 3).

In the very ill it is sometimes impossible to make an accurate diagnosis; but to let a distressing symptom continue in the hope of producing a clear picture can rarely, if ever, be justified. Symptomatic relief must be given, and, when time is short, it may be necessary to produce relief by using several drugs at once rather than one at a time.

Gastrointestinal symptoms

Dry mouth

This may be caused by:

Drugs, especially tricyclic antidepressants, phenothiazines, antihistamines, anticholinergic drugs.
Local radiotherapy.
Mouth breathing.
Anorexia.
Dehydration.

Dry mouth is a common symptom, frequently due to a combination of causes. For example, a patient with liver metastases may have prochlorperazine maleate (Stemetil) 5 mg 4-hourly with his analgesic to control nausea and pain; he may also tend to doze with his mouth open and have a poor appetite, with little stimulation of the salivary glands by the sight and smell of food. It is sometimes possible to alter the drug regimen and to give appropriate drugs to stimulate appetite (see 'Anorexia'). Patients should be encouraged to suck acid sweets or chew gum to increase the flow of saliva. Artificial saliva is occasionally useful and is made up as follows:

Methylcellulose 20   12 g
Lemon essence soluble 0·2 ml
Water to 600 ml

Dilute with an equal volume of water before use.

Intravenous fluids and nasogastric feeding cannot be justified in dying patients. They rarely feel thirsty and it is possible to control the only common symptom of dehydration, namely a dry mouth, by local measure such as frequent small drinks or crushed ice to suck.

Sore mouth

Sore mouth is caused by:

Monilial infection.
Ill-fitting dentures and decaying teeth.
Aphthous ulceration.
Vitamin deficiencies.
Blood dyscrasias.
Methotrexate.

Monilial infection of the mouth is common and causes considerable distress. Predisposing factors include steroid administration and the use of broad-spectrum antibiotics. The attending doctor and nurse should be alert to the need for prevention and early treatment. Oral hygiene is important. If infection occurs, it requires prompt treatment with nystatin oral suspension 100,000 units/ml. The dentures must be removed and the mouth and dentures treated with 1 ml nystatin suspension 4-hourly, until 48 hours after clinical cure. Unfortunately, the infection often recurs and when this happens it is wise to follow the nystatin treatment with amphotericin (Fungilin) lozenges, 1 10-mg tablet twice a day, as a simple means of prophylaxis.

Aphthous ulceration of the mouth is not common. It can be treated with carbenoxolone (Bioral) pellets 5 mg or gel or with hydrocortisone lozenges BPC (Corlan pellets 2·5 mg, 1 four times daily). Vitamin supplements are often given to patients with a sore tongue and angular stomatitis but with rather disappointing results.

Dysphagia

Causes of dysphagia are:

Defeat in the neuromuscular mechanism, e.g. pseudobulbar palsy, cerebellar disorders.
Mechanical obstruction: *intrinsic*, as in carcinoma of oesophagus or be-

nign oesophageal stricture associated with hiatus hernia; or *extrinsic*, as in pressure from enlarged mediastinal lymph nodes.

Psychogenic.

Drugs have little part in the management of dysphagia, though high doses of glucocorticosteroids may cause some shrinkage of enlarged mediastinal nodes. Palliative surgery with the insertion of an oesophageal tube should be considered in patients with an oesophageal carcinoma, unless the prognosis is short (see Chapter 9). Radiotherapy is of value in intrinsic and extrinsic obstruction (see Chapter 7).

Nausea and vomiting

These result from stimulation of the emetic centres in the brain stem by afferent impulses from the gut, cerebral cortex, or the closely related chemo-receptor trigger zone. This stimulation is caused by:

Drugs; e.g. digoxin, morphine, oestrogens.
Biochemical changes; e.g. Uraemia, hypercalcaemia.
Gastric irritation; e.g. carcinoma of stomach.
Intestinal obstruction.
Raised intracranial pressure.

There are a great many causes of vomiting in terminal malignant disease. For some of these the treatment will not differ from that practiced in general medicine, but others present special problems of management in dying patients and these are discussed below.

Hypercalcaemia

This should always be suspected in patients with widespread osteolytic bony metastases, particularly from carcinoma of breast. It may also occur in ectopic parathyroid hormone secretion, mainly associated with carcinoma of the bronchus. It is characterized by weakness, anorexia, nausea and vomiting. The primary treatment is with glucocorticosteroids. If the patient is vomiting, injection of hydrocortisone 100 mg should be given, followed by oral prednisolone 10 mg three times a day, reducing the dose slowly as improvement occurs. In many cases a maintenance dose of prednisolone 10–15 mg/24 h is acceptable to patient and doctor but if long-term steroid treatment is contra-indicated then oral phosphate should be given (Phosphate-Sandoz Effervescent Tablets) 1–2 thrice daily. There is a group of patients with widespread bony metastases who suffer from vomiting which is not well controlled by antiemetics but who do not have demonstrable hypercalcaemia. Their vomiting does, however, respond to the above steroid regimen. One can only label the entity as 'steroid-responsive vomiting', and speculate that it is due to some biochemical abnormality other than hypercalcaemia.

Intestinal Obstruction

This is a fairly common occurrence in the terminal phase of abdominal malignancies and is especially found in ovarian and colorectal cancers. It is usually of slow onset, intermittent at first. Characteristic symptoms at an early stage are bouts of colicky abdominal pain, audible borborygmi, some abdominal distension and diarrhoea. As the obstruction progresses the distension and pain increase, nausea and vomiting start and the bowels become constipated.

There is a widespread fear among doctors and nurses that death from intestinal obstruction is particularly distressing and is accompanied by uncontrollable abdominal pain and vomiting. Such fears may force them into seeking a palliative colostomy for their patient; however, this procedure only adds to distress and it can only be justified in someone with a few months to live (see Chapter 9). At St Christopher's Hospice it has been found possible to gain complete control of the abdominal pain and nausea. The patients may vomit once or twice a day but the final phase need not be distressing. There is little or no place for palliative surgery, nasogastric intubation or intravenous feeding. During the early phases of intestinal obstruction the patient should be given a softening aperient (one that does not induce peristalsis), e.g. dioctyl sodium sulphosuccinate tablets (Dioctyl Forte) 1–2 twice a day. Pain and nausea can be treated orally with analgesics and antiemetics.

If painful colic is a problem, diphenoxylate 2·5 mg with atropine 0·025 mg (Lomotil), 2 tablets four times a day or when needed is helpful. As the obstruction increases the bowels become constipated and the aperient should be discontinued. The patient may continue to tolerate oral medication but will frequently need analgesics and antiemetics by injection or suppository. The latter route is of great value in managing obstructed patients at home—a perfectly feasible proposition—or to avoid frequent intramuscular injections. A useful combination is:

> Oxycodone suppositories (Proladone)* 30 mg 1–2, 8-hourly. Prochlorperazine maleate suppositories (Stemetil) 25 mg 8-hourly.

Many patients put themselves on a fluid diet, but some have the occasional favourite meal; the enjoyment of eating fish and chips, for example, is apparently worth the almost inevitable vomit some hours later.

Although a patient will become dehydrated in his last days, it is possible to relieve the dry mouth—the only distressing symptom—with frequent small drinks and crushed ice to suck.

Raised intracranial pressure

This occurs in patients with cerebral tumours, primary or secondary, and is characterized by headache, blurred vision, nausea and vomiting and, sometimes, local neurological signs and mental confusion. If the patient is elderly or terminal it is probably wise to treat symptomatically with analgesics and antiemetics. However, there are many cases where correction of the raised pressure offers a useful and enjoyable remission to the patient and his family. With treatment he will lose his headache and vomiting, vision and mental state will improve and neurological signs decrease. Dexamethasone tablets should be started in high dosage, 16 mg/24 h. Response usually occurs in 24–48 hours but treatment should be continued for a week at this dosage before assessing the full response. If there is no improvement, the drug should be discontinued. The problem arises when there is a considerable improvement; the doctor and patient are naturally reluctant to reduce the dose

---

* This drug has been temporarily discontinued; morphine suppositories, 15–30 mg 6-hourly, may be used instead.

of such an effective drug but this reluctance should be balanced by the necessity of keeping steroid dosage as low as possible to avoid side-effects.

The decision about dosage will depend on the nature of the tumour. In rapidly advancing disease the risk of long-term steroid effects can be disregarded and the dexamethasone dosage maintained at a high level. If the disease is advancing more slowly, an attempt should be made to reduce the dose of steroids—a suggested pattern is by 2 mg/week. This reduction should continue until either the symptoms recur or an effective maintenance dose is reached at about 2–4 mg/24 h. With a low maintenance dose it is occasionally possible and desirable to increase it again at one step to 16 mg/24 h if the patient deteriorates, but three or four 'resurrections' of patients with expanding cerebral tumours can never be justified.

Dexamethasone is thought to act by suppression of local cerebral inflammation; it has no effect on the tumour cells themselves. Thus as the tumour grows, producing further brain destruction, the patient's symptoms will inevitably return and the doctor will be faced with an extremely difficult decision about the quality of life he is prolonging. The time will come, for example, if the patient is paralysed and very confused, when no useful purpose is served by continuing treatment, and the steroids should be discontinued during the next week or 10 days.

Antiemetics

In many cases of terminal malignant disease there is no further specific treatment for the nausea and vomiting, and antiemetics are required. The useful drugs can be divided into four main groups:

1. *Phenothiazines:* e.g. chlorpromazine (Largactil), prochlorperazine maleate (Stemetil), promazine hydrochloride (Sparine). This is probably the most useful group of drugs; they act on the chemoreceptor zone in the medulla. The antiemetic effect is combined with a tranquillizing action which is of value. Chlorpromazine and prochlorperazine can be given by mouth, in tablet or syrup, by intramuscular injection (i.m.) and by suppository.

2. *Antihistamines:* e.g. cyclizine (Marzine), dimenhydrinate (Dramamine). These act on the vomiting centres; they can be given by tablet and intramuscular injection.

3. *Metoclopramide* (Maxolon). This acts both on the chemoreceptor trigger zone and peripherally, stimulating normal peristalsis and relaxing the pyloric antrum. It may be given by mouth in tablet or syrup, or by intramuscular injection.

4. *Anticholinnergic drugs:* e.g. hyoscine. Hyoscine reduces gut motility and also greatly diminishes secretion of saliva; this second effect reduces the usefulness of hyoscine in the control of nausea and vomiting.

A patient with severe nausea and vomiting will at first need antiemetics parenterally, probably a phenothiazine such as chlorpromazine 25 mg i.m. 4-hourly or prochlorperazine maleate 12·5 mg i.m. immediately and 6·25 mg i.m. 4-hourly. These may be combined with an analgesic if pain is a problem. In the majority of cases the vomiting will settle on this regimen and oral medication can be started with chlorpromazine 25-mg tablets 4-hourly or prochlorperazine maleate tablets 5–10 mg 4-hourly. If a phenothiazine alone does not control symptoms, an additional antiemetic of a different group should be added. Some patients will require three drugs for complete control, such as:

Prochlorperazine tablets	5 mg 4-hourly
Metoclopramide tablets	10 mg three times a day, before meals
Cyclizine tablets	50 mg three times a day

The same principle applies to parenteral control, except that metoclopramide is more effective by mouth, due to its specific effect on the stomach wall.

There are a number of patients who remain unable to tolerate drugs by mouth and where long-term injection control should be avoided, either because of painful injection sites or because home management is required. For this group suppositories of chlorpromazine 50–100 mg 8–hourly or pro-chlorperazine maleate 25 mg 8-hourly should be tried. If diamorphine is required for pain it can be given subcutaneously, with the phenothiazine by suppository, thus sparing intramuscular sites.

Anorexia

This is one of the most common and distressing symptoms, occurring in all types of cancer. Probably the most important remedy is the serving of small portions of attractively prepared food; many patients will comment that they enjoyed and finished a small amount whereas they would not even have attempted a larger helping. They are often put off by traditional invalid fare but would fancy a small tasty serving of kipper, bacon or even jellied eels! A multivitamin tonic or alcohol before meals may help psychologically.

Glucocorticosteroids are the only effective drug treatment of anorexia. Prednisolone tablets 5 mg three times a day is an adequate dose and most patients report an improvement in appetite within a week, sometimes finding that their sense of taste returns first. With this dosage there are few complications; the only serious one is a small risk of gastric bleeding and this is possibly reduced by using the enteric-coated prednisolone tablet. There are no absolute contra-indications but it is usually best to avoid steroids in patients with diabetes, peptic ulceration, tuberculosis and large infected wounds.

Constipation

The majority of patients complain of constipation. This is due to their inactivity, a diet low in roughage, and possibly also to the effect of drugs. These three factors are difficult to alter; bran is often tried but is usually unacceptable in the very ill. The treatment of constipation, with the exception of the group with intestinal obstruction (discussed above), is therefore the correct prescribing of aperients. There are two main types:

1. *Stimulant purgatives*, e.g. senna, bisacodyl (Dulcolax), danthron (as in Dorbanex).

2. *Faecal softeners*, e.g. liquid paraffin, dioctyl sodium sulphosuccinate, methylcellulose, lactulose (Duphalac).

Most patients are best managed with a combination of both types of aperient. If the stimulant type is given alone there will often be painful colic; if the softeners alone are prescribed the patient may develop a loaded rectum with soft faeces making manual evacuation impossible.

A possible combination is dioctyl sodium sulphosuccinate tablets (Dioctyl Forte) 1–2 twice a day and senna (Senokot) 2–4 alternate nights; or a proprietary combined product such as Dorbanex Medo or Forte 5–10 ml once or twice a day (danthron BP and poloxamer). If the patient presents with a loaded rectum and hard faeces, evacuation from below is first required, either by suppository, glycerine or bisacodyl (Dulcolax) or by enema. Sometimes in spite of regular aperients the bowels do not open regularly and a good general rule is for a rectal examination to be performed on the third day, inserting suppositories if the rectum is loaded. Such a regimen will avoid the physical and mental distress of patients who are constipated for a week or more.

Faecal incontinence is more often due to impaction than any other cause.

Paraplegic patients frequently have severe constipation with abdominal distension. They may be helped by either neostigmine bromide tablets (Prostigmin) 15 mg thrice daily, or bethanechol tablets (Myotonine) 10 mg thrice daily.

Diarrhoea

Diarrhoea can be caused by:

Steatorrhoea, particularly in pancreatic insufficiency due to carcinoma of pancreas.
Incomplete intestinal obstruction.
Abdominal or pelvic radiotherapy.
Broad-spectrum antibiotics.
Infections.
Tumours of colon or rectum.

Pancreatic insufficiency

This is common in patients with carcinoma of the head of pancreas. The diarrhoea is characteristic, the stool being bulky, pale and greasy, flushing away only with difficulty. The patient may also complain of wind and abdominal distension. Treatment is with pancreatic replacements, e.g. Pancrex V 1–2 capsules with food. It is important to emphasize to the patient that he needs this with each meal or snack.

Antidiarrhoeal drugs

The two antidiarrhoeal drugs commonly used are codeine phosphate tablets 15–60 mg three times a day and diphenoxylate with atropine (Lomotil) 1–2 tablets four times a day. Both are effective and may be used in combination in severe cases.

Rectal discharge

This is a considerable problem in patients with colorectal carcinoma for which only a palliative colostomy has been performed. The anal sphincter is often unable to control the discharge which leaks through, causing distress. If the patient is fairly well, a course of local palliative radiotherapy may be indicated (see Chapter 7). This symptom is often improved by a course of prednisolone sodium phosphate (Predsol) retention enemas—one being given every 24 hours, preferably at night, with the foot of the bed tipped up. Predsol suppositories are more convenient but probably less effective.

Hiccough

This occurs in patients with uraemia and diseases of the stomach and abdomen. The two most effective drugs are chlorpromazine (Largactil) tablets 25 mg 4-hourly or when required, and metoclopramide (Maxolon) tablets 10 mg three times a day or when required.

Itch

Itch is found in many patients with obstructive jaundice due to the accumulation of bile acids. Cholestyramine (Cuemid, Questran) is an exchange resin which binds bile acids in the bowel and thus prevents their absorption. One or two sachets daily are usually effective, but they are rather unpalatable for the very ill.

Antihistamines orally may relieve itch, probably due to their mild sedative effect. Crotamiton (Eurax) and topical steroids are useful local antipruritic agents.

Respiratory symptoms

Dyspnoea, cough and chest pain are the three common respiratory symptoms.

Dyspnoea

Dyspnoea literally means 'difficult breathing' and the term is used to refer to a state in which the patient is conscious of having to make an effort to breathe. The feeling of breathlessness arises in most people when ventilation rises to about 40 per cent of maximum breathing capacity. The causes of dyspnoea may be summarized as follows.

Increased ventilatory demand

1. Raised basal metabolic rate; e.g. fever, hyperthyroidism.
2. Metabolic acidosis; e.g. uraemia, diabetic ketosis.
3. Anaemia.

These are not often the chief factors in producing dyspnoea in terminal malignancy, but they are frequently found in association with other causes.

Decreased ventilatory capacity

1. *Airway obstruction*, which may be:
(a) *Upper respiratory tract obstruction* including the trachea and main bronchi. This may be caused by tumours of the pharynx, larynx and thyroid or by enlarged cervical or mediastinal lymph nodes. It is characterized by stridor.

(*b*) *Intrapulmonary obstruction*. Chronic bronchitis and asthma are often found in association with carcinoma of the bronchus. It is characterized by wheeze.

2. *Loss of lung elasticity* due to emphysema or pulmonary fibrosis including postirradiation fibrosis.

3. *Loss of functioning lung tissue* due to:
   Compression, e.g., in pleural effusion or pneumonothorax
   Pulmonary oedema from cardiac failure or lymphangitis carcinomatosa
   Pneumonias
   Lung tumours, primary or secondary

4. *Respiratory muscle weakness* in paraplegics with intercostal paralysis.

It will be self-evident that there are a great many causes of dyspnoea in the terminally ill. For many of them—for example, cardiac failure—the treatment will not differ from that used in general medicine. However, the management of some causes of dyspnoea in dying patients presents special problems, and a distinctive approach is needed.

Anaemia

A high proportion of patients with advanced malignant disease are anaemic; but in few cases is the anaemia due to iron deficiency or other correctable factors, and the physician is often faced with the question of whether to transfuse.

In the majority of cases the anaemia is only part of a widespread disease process and does not in itself produce many symptoms; transfusion may be distressing to the patient and may fail to produce any worthwhile improvement. Transfusion should probably only be considered prior to further active treatment—for example, by chemotherapy—or in the rare circumstance where a short-lasting improvement would be of real benefit to the patient and his family—for example, some important family event.

Mediastinal tumours

These are usually lymph node metastases from carcinomas (especially of the bronchus and breast) or nodes involved by Hodgkin's disease or the non-Hodgkin lymphomas. The clinical effects result from compression of normal structures and are predictable: compression of the trachea and main bronchi causes dyspnoea and stridor, compression of the oesophagus produces dysphagia and of the superior vena cava (SVC) produces the syndrome of SVC obstruction. Involvement of the phrenic nerve may produce diaphragmatic paralysis, of the left recurrent laryngeal nerve may produce hoarseness, and of the sympathetic trunk may produce Horner's syndrome.

Treatment will obviously depend on the site of origin of the tumour and will probably involve radiotherapy with or without cytotoxic drugs and hormone manipulation. However, many patients who present with dyspnoea due to mediastinal obstruction are very ill and immediate relief is required. This is best obtained by using high doses of glucocorticosteroids such as dexamethasone tablets 4 mg four times a day. This often produces shrinkage of nodes and a rapid clinical improvement. The patient may thus become fit enough for further, more specific, treatment and the dose of steroids can be slowly reduced.

Chronic bronchitis and asthma

Many patients who develop carcinoma of the bronchus do so with a background of chronic obstructive lung disease. Secondary or intrinsic asthma will frequently be associated with the chronic bronchitis.

The treatment of chronic bronchitis and asthma at this stage differs somewhat from that practiced in general medicine. The antispasmodic group of drugs remain useful: for example, salbutamol (Ventolin) tablets 2–4 mg three times a day and aminophylline, especially by suppository, benefits many patients. Sodium cromoglycate (Intal) has not been found of benefit and is difficult for the very ill to manage as it is given as an inhalant.

Glucocorticosteroids are by far the most effective drugs and, in patients with only a short prognosis, they can obviously be given without fear of long-term side-effects. Prednisolone tablets 10 mg thrice daily should be started and given for at least a week before slow reduction is attempted to a maintenance dose of 5 mg two or three times a day.

In cases of severe dyspnoea with bronchospasm and in lymphangitis carcinomatosa it may be wise to start at once with an injection of hydrocortisone 100 mg or the more potent glucocorticosteroid, dexamethasone, reducing steroid dosage as before. Patients with chronic bronchitis and asthma are prone to chest infections, which are treated with antibiotics and physiotherapy if this is thought appropriate (see below).

Pleural effusion

Aspiration of pleural fluid may be necessary to establish the diagnosis and, in fairly fit patients, the tapping of an effusion with the instillation of cytotoxic drugs can produce a worthwhile remission (see Chapter 8). However, there is little place for pleural aspiration in the care of the terminally ill; they often find the procedure distressing and the effusion usually builds up to the same level within a few days so that no lasting benefit is obtained.

Pneumonia

The treatment of chest infections is one of the most emotive issues in this field. Hospice doctors are often asked, 'Do you treat pneumonia?' as if there was a firm policy laid down which was rigidly applied to all patients. Each case must be carefully and individually considered. It would, for example, be as inappropriate to give antibiotics by injection and physiotherapy to a virtually moribund patient as it would be to withhold such treatment from one with a prognosis of some months who needed to settle business affairs or hopefully to come to terms with dying. The physician's judgement will be based on an imponderable factor—the quality of life offered. Guidelines in assessing this will be the patient's age and family ties, his general condition and prognosis and—in particular—his respiratory capacity, bearing in mind that each succeeding chest infection will lower his vital capacity. It is often wise to treat a patient actively when first admitted to hospital so as to give the staff time to get to know him and his family and to help their particular needs.

Doctors should remember that in many cases the use of opiates to relieve pain, cough and dyspnoea is the right and appropriate treatment for a chest infection in a dying patient, whereas antibiotics would often be inappropriate. If a decision to use antibiotics is made they should be employed in normal dosage for 7–10 days. Amoxycillin, co-trimoxazale (Septrin) and chloramphenicol are all used at standard doses; the last is especially valuable since resistance is not often found and the rare blood dyscrasias can be disregarded. Physiotherapy to the chest should be given.

The use of oxygen

Oxygen therapy is sometimes useful until other medication is effective in a patient who becomes acutely breathless. It does not continue to help the chronic dyspnoea of terminally ill patients and the presence of an oxygen mask and cylinder is distressing to dying patients and their families. Better control of dyspnoea can be obtained from the correct use of the opiates and other drugs.

The use of opiates

There will come a time when specific treatment is no longer effective—the mediastinal lymph nodes are growing in spite of radiotherapy and glucocorticosteroids; the pleural effusion reaccumulates a few days after aspiration; pulmonary oedema no longer resolves with digoxin and diuretics. In all these cases, and in many others, the appropriate line of treatment will be the use of opiates.

Opiates relieve dyspnoea by diminishing the sensitivity of the respiratory centre to increased carbon dioxide tension in the blood. There is a decrease in minute volume due to a decrease in both the rate and depth of breathing. Traditionally, doctors have been warned against using opiates for patients in respiratory distress; statements such as 'Opiates must never be used in asthmatic patients' and 'Morphine is dangerous in all patients with respiratory insufficiency' are to be found in standard textbooks. Such statements are, of course, correct when applied to patients with remediable illness. But they must not prevent doctors using the most valuable drugs at their disposal for the relief of dyspnoea, perhaps the most distressing symptom of the dying.

The dose of diamorphine or morphine used should be titrated against the patient's response, as outlined in Chapter 5, an attempt being made to find the lowest dose which will relieve symptoms. Diamorphine 5 mg 4-hourly would be a suitable starting dose, but much higher doses may be needed. The patient will probably tolerate his medication orally, in an elixir of diamorphine with prochlorperazine maleate 5 mg (Stemetil) or chlorpromazine (Largactil) 12·5–25 mg to potentiate the effect and to act as a tranquillizer. In the very ill it may be necessary to give diamorphine and a tranquillizer by intramuscular injection.

The doctor is occasionally presented with an extremely ill dyspnoeic patient whose symptoms have been inadequately controlled over the preceding days and weeks. He is then in a quandary. He has the choice of leaving the patient in pain and gasping for breath or of giving an adequate dose of an opiate, knowing that it may markedly depress the respiratory centre and hasten the patient's death. It is obviously a difficult decision to make but he should remember that to relieve the distress of dying has always been accepted as correct medicine.

The use of hyoscine

Hyoscine (scopolamine) is an anticholinergic drug related to atropine, having a number of actions:

1. it dries up secretions of all exocrine glands;
2. it relaxes smooth muscle;
3. it is a CNS depressant (unlike atropine which is a stimulant);
4. it may, however, confuse the elderly.

These actions make hyoscine an excellent drug to abolish the so-called 'death rattle'. This is caused by an accumulation of bronchial secretions in a patient too weak to cough. It is extremely distressing to a watching family and others in the ward, though not usually to the patient himself, who may be semiconscious. Injection hyoscine 0·4–0·6 mg should be given; if the patient is not having an opiate already to control pain or dyspnoea then diamorphine 5–10 mg is added to increase sedation and to prevent the occasional excitement. The drug may be repeated 4-hourly but it is preferable to avoid more than three doses in 24-hours as tolerance to hyoscine occurs.

Cough

Cough may be conveniently classified into dry and productive, as the causes vary.

Dry cough
External irritants especially smoke and dust.
Pressure on a bronchus from primary or metastatic tumour.
Early acute bronchitis with mucosal inflammation.

Productive cough
Generalized, as in chronic bronchitis
Localized—Pheumonia
          Lung abscess
          Neoplasm
Obviously the ideal treatment of cough is directed at removing the cause: stopping smoking, the use of antibiotics for acute bronchitis and pneumonia, surgery or radiotherapy for neoplasm. However, curative treatment is not possible in many cases, and the patient may request the treatment of his cough. In general terms it is reasonable to suppress a dry cough, but a productive cough should be allowed to continue unless it is very exhausting and is disturbing sleep.

Antitussives

Antitussives act at two sites: on the respiratory mucosa and on the cough centre in the medulla.

Local action

On inspired air. The most effective means is to stop the patient smoking! The inspiration of warm, moist air will often relieve a hacking cough; this may be achieved with a steam kettle or humidifier, or the use of benzoin inhalation BPC.

Expectorants. These are claimed to stimulate the cough and make it more effective by causing an increase in bronchial secretions—for example, ammonia and ipececuanha mixture BPC. They are not of proven efficacy.

Mucolytics. Bromhexine (Bisolvon) 8 mg is a drug which reduces the viscosity of bronchial secretions by breaking up the long protein fibres; it therefore makes expectoration easier. It can be given as a tablet 8 mg 1–2 thrice daily or in liquid form (8 mg in 10 ml).

Decongestants. A great many proprietary preparations are made up to include a decongestant such as pseudoephedrine, often combined with an antihistamine and codeine—for example, Actifed Compound Linctus, Phensedyl Cough Linctus. These are widely prescribed and appear to help many patients.

Central action

   Codeine linctus or pholcodeine linctus
   Methadone linctus
   Diamorphine linctus

These are listed in ascending order of potency and should usually be tried in this order. Methadone and diamorphine are also respiratory depressants.

   In practice, a combination of antitussive agents is often used; for example:
   bromhexine (Bisolvon) tablets 8 mg thrice daily and codeine linctus 10 ml at night; or
   diphendydramine hydrochloride BP 14 mg with ammonium chloride BP 135 mg (Benylin Expectorant) 5 ml four times a day and methadone linctus 10 ml at night.

Chest pain

This is the third of the triad of respiratory symptoms and requires only brief mention in this chapter. The treatment is threefold: palliative radiotherapy if appropriate, and if the patient is well enough (see Chapter 7); intercostal block (see Chapter 5); lastly, analgesics in adequate dosage (see Chapter 5).

Urinary symptoms

Frequency and incontinençe

These symptoms are often found in patients with advanced malignant disease, and can cause great distress. 'I don't mind what happens to me as long as I don't become incontinent' expresses a sentiment that is commonly felt.

   In order to offer the appropriate treatment it is important to know the common causes of these symptoms.

Polyuria

Polyuria may be due to:

1. Diabetes mellitus
2. Diabetes insipidus—from a primary or secondary tumour involving the posterior pituitary gland, or following hypophysectomy.
3. Chronic renal failure.
4. Functional—from excessive drinking.

The treatment of these conditions does not differ from that practised in general medicine.

Neurological causes

Neurological causes include:

1. Any tumour causing paraplegia by pressure on the spinal cord or affecting the cauda equina with characteristic saddle anaesthesia. Immediate radiotherapy and/or a decompression laminectomy should be considered if the patient is well enough.
2. Cerebral tumours and cerebral arteriosclerosis.

Pelvic disease

This includes intrapelvic malignancy (e.g. arising from bladder, prostate, uterus, pelvic colon), benign prostate hypertrophy and postirradiation bladder damage.

Urinary infections

In cases of urinary infection the frequency will usually be associated with painful micturition. The urine should be cultured for micro-organisms and a full course of an appropriate antibiotic given. Frequently, however, the infection is associated with a structural abnormality of the urinary tract and recurs after treatment.

Emepronium (Cetiprin)

This is an anticholinergic drug similar to propantheline though said to have its greatest effect on the urinary bladder, increasing bladder capacity and therefore delaying the desire to void. It is useful in all types of urinary frequency if specific treatment directed to the cause is not possible or is ineffective. It should be used with caution in cases of bladder neck obstruction as it may precipitate retention.

A usual dose of emepronium is 100–200 mg thrice daily, or 200 mg at night if the frequency is only at night.

Catheterization

This procedure should be considered in all terminally ill patients with severe frequency or incontinence which cannot be controlled by specific measures.

The usual risks associated with long-term catheterization do not apply here, and for a great majority of patients it is the most satisfactory means of controlling a distressing problem. If possible, the procedure should be discussed with the patient a few days beforehand, for there will always be a few who prefer either a condom or incontinence padding.

A self-retaining catheter should be passed under full aseptic conditions; in most patients this is quite painless. For difficult catheterization—for example, in patients with huge carcinomas of the vulva or cervix, in prostatic carcinoma and in particularly anxious patients—it is helpful to give intravenous diazepam (Valium) 10 mg a few minutes beforehand.

It is, of course, impossible to maintain sterile urine in a patient with an indwelling catheter; but this does not matter in the terminally ill as the risk of late chronic pyelonephritis can be ignored. What will cause distress to the patient is an acute bladder infection producing suprapubic pain or a blockage of the catheter by debris.

The following regimen has been followed at St Christopher's Hospice for some years, and has produced a marked decrease in catheter problems. The catheter is inserted under aseptic conditions and changed monthly—or 6-monthly if a Silastic catheter is used. An adequate fluid intake is encouraged.

Co-trimoxazole (Septrin) tablets, 2 twice daily are given for 2 days on catheterization and recatheterization. (Co-trimoxazole is bactericidal for bacteria accidentally introduced during the procedure.) The patient is maintained on a urinary antiseptic—not an antibiotic or sulphonamide to which resistance will soon develop. Hexamine mandelate (Mandelamine) 0·5 g 2 tablets four times a day can be given or, more conveniently, hexamine hippurate (Hiprex) 1 g twice daily. The latter has a wide antibacterial spectrum and bacterial resistance is alleged not to occur.

In the few cases where an acute urinary infection occurs in spite of these measures, the appropriate antibiotic should be given for a full course.

In patients unable to swallow tablets a daily bladder wash-out should be given using chlorhexidine gluconate solution (Hibitane) 1 in 5000. Noxytiolin bladder instillations (Noxyflex) 1 twice daily for 2 days are useful if wash-outs are ineffective.

Urinary retention

This is a much less common problem, which may be caused by:

1. Drugs especially anticholinergic drugs, propantheline (Pro-Banthine), sympathomimetic drugs (ephedrine, which is a component of some treatments for asthma), and tricyclic antidepressants. These drugs probably only precipitate retention in patients who already have some degree of bladder neck obstruction.

2. Neurological causes (as for incontinence).

3. Bladder neck obstruction or urethral obstruction, e.g. carcinoma of bladder, cervix or prostate, benign prostate hypertrophy.

In neurological cases it is worth trying bethanechol chloride (Myotonine) 5 mg subcutaneously for acute retention, or 10 mg thrice daily for chronic cases.

Occasionally, this may avoid the need for catheterization. In most patients a catheter is required and the same routine should be applied as for incontinent patients. There are a few cases where catheterization under general anaesthetic is required; suprapubic drainage is almost never necessary.

Central nervous system symptoms

Depression

Visitors to hospices, or to a home where a dying patient is being well cared for, are often surprised that the atmosphere is far from depressing. Most patients face a severe or terminal illness with remarkable courage and cheerfulness; this is especially true if their physical needs such as pain and anorexia are controlled, they have honest communication with their families and medical attendants, and spiritual help if desired.

Thus, if a doctor attends a dying patient who appears depressed, his main attention should be given to relieving physical, mental and spiritual distress.

There remains a group, especially those whose illness is protracted or who have an unsupportive family, who develop clinical depression. These may be helped by the tricyclic antidepressants such as amitriptyline (Tryptizol) 25–50 mg at night or dothiepin (Prothiaden) 25–50 mg at night. It has been found that the higher dosage more commonly given in psychiatric practices can cause confusion in the dying. This is probably due to their potentiation by the phenothiazines which are often prescribed for their antiemetic action or to potentiate opiates.

The monoamine oxidase inhibitors are best avoided because of their interaction with certain types of food and many drugs. Electroconvulsive therapy (ECT) is almost never required (see Chapter 4).

Anxiety

Although drugs have a definite role in the management of anxiety in the dying, the most important therapeutic tool is TIME—time spent by the patient with his doctor in which he can voice without embarrassment his fears for the future; time supporting the family, helping with practical and emotional problems; time with priest, social worker and others who can help. Many of these aspects are discussed elsewhere—see Chapters 4, 10, 11.

Drugs should be an addition to time given and not as a substitute. The two useful groups are the phenothiazines such as chlorpromazine (Largactil) and the benzodiazepines such as diazepam (Valium). There is not a great deal to choose between these groups, though some individual patients seem to do better on one than the other.

If the patient is also nauseated, then a phenothiazine would be the obvious choice: chlorpromazine (Largactil) 10–25 mg thrice daily or promazine hydrochloride (Sparine) 25–50 mg thrice daily. If the patient is receiving a mild phenothiazine such as prochlorperazine maleate (Stemetil) 5 mg 4-hourly with an elixir diamorphine for pain, it would be logical to change to a stronger tranquillizer such as chlorpromazine (Largactil) 12·5–25 mg 4-hourly. Otherwise, diazepam (Valium) 2–5 mg thrice daily or chlordiazepoxide (Librium) 5–10 mg thrice daily can be prescribed.

Insomnia

Many patients with terminal illness suffer with insomnia due to unrelieved physical or mental symptoms such as pain, anxiety or nocturnal frequency. Insomnia improves as these are relieved.

If hypnotics are required, the benzodiazepines are probably the first choice; they induce more normal sleep and are safe even if a high dose is taken. Nitrazepam (Mogadon) 5–10 mg at night or diazepam (Valium) 5–10 mg at night are suitable. Occasionally the benzodiazepines seem to confuse the elderly and dichloralphenazone (Welldorm), a chloral derivative, 650–1300 mg at night is preferred; this can be given as 1–2 tablets or 15–30 ml syrup.

In an elderly patient who is already confused, chlormethiazole (Heminevrin) is a useful drug both for daytime sedation and as an hypnotic; the dosage is 500 mg thrice daily and 1000 mg at night. It is made as a large tablet or syrup; unfortunately, both are rather unpalatable.

Some cases of insomnia are due to an underlying depression which should be treated as suggested in Chapter 4. There will always be some patients who have taken barbiturates happily for many years to promote sleep, and these should be continued if the patient requests it.

Night sweats are an occasional cause of insomnia and are distressing to the patient, especially if he is at home and changes of night clothes and bedding are required. They often respond to indomethacin (Indocid) given at night, either 100 mg suppository or 25–50 mg tablet.

Confusion

The differential diagnosis and management of confusion in a terminally ill patient is one of the most difficult problems that a doctor concerned with the dying has to face. In addition, the family are usually greatly distressed, feeling that meaningful communication with a relative may no longer be possible. It is important to have in mind several possible causes:

1. *Drugs*, especially excessive doses of tranquillizers and analgesics, tricyclic antidepressants or alcohol.
2. *Biochemical causes:* Uraemia; anoxia; hypoglycaemia.
3. *Toxic* from infections such as pneumonia.
4. *Postepileptic.*
5. *Cerebral tumours*, primary or secondary.
6. *Other causes of cerebral damage*, especially cerebral arteriosclerosis.
7. *Psychogenic*, e.g. altered environment, especially in the elderly.

From such a list, which is not exhaustive, it is apparent that specific treatment can be attempted in a certain proportion of cases; chest infections treated, excess sedation decreased, the dose of insulin or oral hypoglycaemic drugs reduced to match the patient's diminished food intake. It is sometimes difficult to help the dyspnoeic patient with chronic obstructive lung disease and to find the dose of an opiate which will relieve his distress and yet not precipitate anoxic confusion, especially at night. Many confused patients will respond to a familiar face or voice, or a sympathetic nurse with time to sit and listen.

Cerebral tumours

A proportion of patients with cerebral tumours develop epileptic fits, and it is extremely important to control these, as even in an unconscious patient they are frightening to the family. Anticonvulsants should not be given prophylactically in all cases of brain tumour; but once a fit has occurred the patient should start on phenytoin sodium (Epanutin) 100 mg thrice daily if he is able to take tablets. If this proves inadequate, phenobarbitone 30–60 mg twice daily should be added and this regimen continued while oral medication is possible. When parenteral drugs are required, due to vomiting or inability to swallow, intramuscular phenobarbitone 60–120 mg twice a day is almost always adequate; it is rare that the bulky phenytoin injections (250 mg in 5 ml) two or three times a day are also needed. Status epilepticus is a rare occurrence. It should be treated with intravenous diazepam (Valium) given slowly at 10 mg/minute.

The use of high dosage adrenocorticosteroids such as dexamethasone in cerebral tumours has already been discussed (p. 102).

It may be justified to give this treatment as a therapeutic trial in a patient suspected of having cerebral metastases who has a malignancy which is likely to spread to the brain, and who presents with confusion and headache. It is often not practicable to arrange for a brain scan, and dexamethasone 16 mg/day can be given for a week to assess the response and thus perhaps establish the diagnosis.

Tranquillizers

It is important to realize that although tranquillizers may make confused patients less aggressive and more amenable to management, they cannot restore mental function deranged by disease. There are therefore a great many confused patients who, in their own way, are fairly happy and who need no psychotrophic drugs.

It is the restless and aggressive confused who need treatment, and probably a monitored dose of an appropriate phenothiazine is the best drug. Thioridazine (Melleril) 25 mg thrice daily is especially suitable for the elderly; but chlorpromazine (Largactil) and promazine hydrochloride (Sparine) are also useful and have the advantage that they can be given by intramuscular injection if required.

The most potent phenothiazine is methotrimeprazine (Nozinan) which is approximately twice as strong as chlorpromazine; it is invaluable in the management of restless dying patients who are inadequately controlled by chlorpromazine. It is usually given 25–50 mg 4-hourly in combination with diamorphine and sometimes with diazepam (Valium) 5–10 mg 4-hourly as well.

Chlormethiazole (Heminevrin) can be used for the elderly confused, both by night and day (500 mg thrice daily and 1000 mg at night).

Local care of fungating tumours

Breast cancer is the commonest neoplasm to cause fungation, but open lesions can also occur with other tumours, both primary and secondary (see Chapter 2). Fungating growths may be painful and they are always distressing to the patient.

The use of local radiotherapy and cytotoxic drugs is discussed in Chapters 7 and 8.

A seven-day course of an appropriate broad-spectrum antibiotic will often temporarily reduce local sepsis and the offensive smell it causes. However, in the majority of cases local applications are the only possible continuing treatment. A great number of preparations are used, and the success of each depends considerably on the enthusiasm of the nurse and the time she is able to give.

Regular cleansing of the area is of prime importance. Eusol diluted with an equal volume of water is excellent to clean heavily infected areas, but in some very sensitive sites such as the vulva, frequent wash-downs with 1 in 2000 chlorhexidine gluconate solution (Hibitane) are all that is tolerated. After cleansing, various soothing dressings are used. Eusol 50 per cent with liquid paraffin 50 per cent or a more dilute solution can be applied, gauze or old linen being soaked in this and then spread out over the lesion, often with the nurse using sterile gloves rather than forceps.

Providone-Iodine 4 per cent (Betadine Skin Cleanser) is also used; it is a powerful non-irritant germicidal agent, does not sting and local sensitivity is rare. An antibiotic spray such as Polybactrin* is probably less effective. If the area is dry and crusted it would be preferable to omit the eusol and paraffin, to cleanse with normal saline if necessary and apply a non-adhesive dressing.

If there is persistent capillary bleeding from the tumour, a non-adhesive dressing should be applied and covered with gauze soaked in 1 in 1000 adrenaline. This will soak through to the wound and yet enable the dressing to be changed without inducing further bleeding.

Barrier preparations such as Kerogel are useful in the perineal area.

Occasionally, in spite of these measures, there is a persistent problem of smell, embarrassing to the patient and his family. Denidor pads, which are incorporated into the dressing, are available for hospital use. An 'Airwick' or deodorizing fans are also effective.

Reference and further reading

GOODMAN, L. S. and GILMAN, A. (Eds.) (1975). *The Pharmacological Basis of Therapeutics*. Macmillan; New York. Balliere Tindall; London.

LAURENCE, D. R. (1973). *Clinical Pharmacology*, Churchill Livingstone; Edinburgh and London.

MODELL, W. (1961). *Relief of Symptoms*. C. V. Mosbey; St Louis.

NIGHTINGALE, Florence (1946). *The Art of Nursing*. Claud Morris; London.

---

* Neomycin sulphate, bacitracin zinc plus polymyxin B sulphate.

The following are the main symptoms on admission of 607 patients admitted with terminal cancer during 1976.

Table 6.1.

Symptom	Percentage*		
	Male	Female	Both
Pain	61·5	69·5	66·0
Anorexia	65·5	58·0	61·75
Weight loss	64·0	55·5	59·75
Cough	53·0	44·5	48·75
Constipation	48·5	43·0	45·75
Dyspnoea	50·0	32·0	41·0
Vomiting and nausea	38·0	43·75	41·0
Effusion and/or oedema	25·0	28·0	26·5
Insomnia	30·0	17·75	23·75
Pressure sores	23·0	20·0	21·5
Weakness	15·75	25·0	20·5
Incontinence	17·75	21·5	19·5
Dysphagia	19·0	13·0	16·0
Cachexia	12·5	10·75	11·5
Drowsiness	12·0	6·75	9·5
Haemorrhage	9·0	7·75	8·5
Jaundice	10·0	5·0	7·5
Colostomy	6·0	7·5	6·75
Paralysis	6·5	3·25	5·0
Diarrhoea	2·5	7·0	4·75
Fistula	1·0	2·25	1·5

* Rounded off to nearest 0·25%.

The following is the result of a survey carried out by three visitors who were asked to assess the control of some major symptoms. They were a doctor on a two-week course and two medical students on electives. This was a random sample of the patients in the wards while these visitors were at St Christopher's Hospice. Nearly all these symptoms are satisfactorily controlled as illustrated above, but this requires constant vigilance on the part of all staff and continual changes of medication.

Note by the Recorder
On reading the case notes of all the patients, I gain the impression that, in the great majority of cases, the symptoms on admission are brought under control.   B. Joan Haram

Symptoms reported in 50 patients on admission (1977)

	Total	Very satisfactory	Satisfactory	Unsatisfactory
Nausea and vomiting	34	20	13	1
Dyspnoea	13	2	11	0
Cough	15	4	10	1
Micturition trouble	10	1	8	1

Definitions
Very satisfactory: symptoms disappeared totally.
Satisfactory: symptom present occasionally and/or patient no longer distressed by it.
Unsatisfactory: symptom present most of the time and patient distressed by it.

7

Radiotherapy in Terminal Care
Thelma D. Bates

The last few weeks of a patient's life are usually a time when active treatment has ceased. Palliative radiotherapy can, however, be helpful during this period provided it is applied skilfully. If misapplied, it can be harmful. The purpose of such palliative radiotherapy must be to relieve distressing symptoms quickly and thus improve the quality of the remaining life. Radiotherapy is not, at this stage, aimed at anticipating symptoms which may never arise, nor in prolonging life though both may be a secondary result of successful treatment. There are rare occasions when radiotherapy may be used to prevent an impending complication such as paraplegia from a collapsing vertebra.

General principles of palliative radiotherapy

These principles are dictated by the limited expectation of life and the need to avoid causing the patient additional discomfort. At no time is good clinical judgement more important. The radiotherapist must be able to make a correct assessment of the situation with the minimum of time-consuming investigations. He must also know what he can reasonably hope to achieve with treatment and what is impossible.

If radiotherapy is indicated it should be given without delay: there is no time to go on to a waiting list. Nor should time be spent on numerous visits to the radiotherapy department. Effective palliation can sometimes be achieved in a single treatment but more often involves the patient in a course of five or six treatments spread over a period of 2 or 3 weeks. Daily treatments protracted over a period of several weeks are not appropriate. Palliative radiotherapy at this stage of the disease should have few or no side-effects, and the benefits of treatment must be carefully balanced against the price the patient has to pay in terms of the time and trouble involved.

There are occasions when radiotherapy can be actually harmful at this stage of the disease. This applies particularly when a tumour is infiltrating a neighbouring structure such as the bladder, bowel or bronchus, when there is a very real risk that radiotherapy, even at palliative dosages, may lead to fistula formation: the symptoms which follow will be even more distressing than those caused by the untreated tumour. On a similar basis, it may be unwise to irradiate the pelvis of a patient dying from uraemia associated with advanced pelvic cancer; the relief of ureteric obstruction may keep the patient alive long enough for her to develop much more distressing terminal symptoms such as severe pelvic pain and an offensive vaginal discharge. Cerebral metastases may be better left untreated in a patient with rapidly progressing, disseminated bronchial carcinoma.

It is not always easy for a radiotherapist to refuse treatment to a patient who is terminally ill. Very often he has known the patient for years and has helped him in the past, and both the patient and his relatives may beg him to help once again. In addition, a radiotherapist may be pressed to treat a patient by his medical colleagues, who themselves have nothing more to offer but who wish to give some positive help. On the other hand, a radiotherapist who feels he can help a patient may be faced by medical or (more often) nursing colleagues, who seek to protect the patient from further therapeutic interference. In all cases, a radiotherapist must be clear in his own mind what he can hope to achieve by treatment. Although he will take psychological factors into consideration, he must be motivated by the possible physical benefit to his patient. Occasionally, a radiotherapist may be asked to 'pretend to treat' a patient, but this unnecessary deception is never justified.

Three factors influence the potential value of radiotherapy in terminal patients. They are the likely radiosensitivity of the tumour itself, the radiotolerance of the surrounding normal tissues, and the degrees to which these tissues have been irradiated in the past. All tissues, both normal and malignant, vary in their response to irradiation and there is a limit to the total dose which tissues will tolerate, even over a period of months or years. Some tumours are very radiosensitive. These include many of the malignant lymphomas, seminomas, nephroblastomas and the rare dysgerminoma of the ovary. On the other hand, some tumours are generally resistant to radiotherapy and are unlikely to respond to palliative dosage. These include most of the bone and soft tissue sarcomas, the cerebral gliomas and malignant melanoma. Squamous cell carcinomas are moderately radiosensitive and adenocarcinomas, particularly those of the gastrointestinal tract, rather less so.

Of the normal tissues, the gastrointestinal tract is one of the most radiosensitive. Large volume irradiation of the abdomen can be expected to cause nausea and diarrhoea, and even small volume palliative radiotherapy, when delivered to the region of the epigastrium or upper lumbar vertebrae, will often cause nausea or vomiting. Most patients and many doctors believe that radiotherapy is invariably associated with distressing nausea and vomiting, but this is not so. Quite wide field irradiation of the chest, head or limbs is well tolerated and is likely to be associated with no more than a sense of tiredness for a few hours after each treatment.

Relief of pain

Palliative radiotherapy has an important part to play in the relief of pain from bone metastases, most commonly those from a primary breast or bronchial carcinoma. A single treatment delivering 1000 rads to a painful metastasis in a limb bone or rib is often sufficient to relieve pain within 7–14 days. In an efficiently run department this can be given on the same day that the patient is seen. Painful metastases in the bony pelvis or in a vertebra will necessitate a fractionated course of treatment in order to keep side-effects to a minimum. Usually a maximum tumour dose of 2000–2500 rads can be delivered in a course of five treatments spread out over 2 weeks. When metastases in the region of the upper lumbar vertebrae are irradiated, an intramuscular injection of prochlorperazine (12·5 mg) given at approximately 20 minutes before treatment will help to prevent nausea and vomiting. Irradiation of a collapsing cervical or dorsal vertebra is worth considering, even if it is not causing pain, as a prophylactic measure against possible incontinence and paralysis.

The bone and joint pain of patients in the late stages of leukaemia often respond to irradiation in both adults and children. During their periods of hospitalization, doses of a few hundred rads can be given to the painful zones on a day-to-day basis as necessary.

Palliative irradiation can sometimes be given to achieve an indirect effect. The painful joints of a patient suffering from hypertrophic pulmonary osteoarthropathy can occasionally be relieved by irradiating a previously untreated primary bronchial carcinoma. In the same way, itching due to jaundice can be relieved by low dose irradiation of hepatic metastases provided they are from a very radiosensitive tumour.

Nerve root pain due to vertebral collapse, and the severe pain of nerve plexus involvement due to advanced breast, gynaecological or colorectal carcinoma, are much more difficult to control by radiotherapy. Irradiation for pain resulting from rib erosion by bronchial carcinoma is also often unrewarding. Analgesic drugs and nerve blocking procedures play a much more important role in these situations.

Control of bleeding

The presence of severe bleeding can be very disturbing to a patient and a short course of radiotherapy to the chest or pelvis can be used to relieve haemoptysis, haematuria or vaginal bleeding, at least temporarily. A simple technique of opposed fields of suitable size can deliver a maximum tumour dose of 2500 rads in five or six treatments at the rate of two treatments per week. As an alternative, bleeding from a vaginal vault recurrence may be controlled by a single insertion of radium. This necessitates admission to the ward for a day or two but does not usually require a general anaesthetic. In a radiotherapy department with a Cathetron or other after-loading machine capable of delivering high intensity irradiation in a matter of minutes rather than hours, this treatment can be given on an out-patient basis.

Control of fungation

One of the problems of radiotherapy is to deliver an adequate dose to the tumour without irreparably damaging the adjacent normal tissues, and it is therefore less of a problem to treat tumours of the surface of the body. Patients are not infrequently seen with disseminated carcinomatosis associated with a primary breast tumour which is either fungating or about to fungate. When time permits, a previously unirradiated tumour, even if quite large, can often be controlled (with healing of ulceration) by a few doses of irradiation. However, if a fungating breast tumour has been irradiated previously, other forms of treatment such as hormone or chemotherapy may be more appropriate.

Using opposed fields of supervoltage radiotherapy aimed tangentially across the breast, a maximum tumour dose of 3500 rads delivered in six treatments at the rate of two treatments per week will control such a tumour just as well as any more protracted technique of daily treatments. In elderly, frail or very sick patients a similar arrangement of fields can be used to deliver a single treatment of 800 rads. If the patient is well enough, this treatment can be repeated a week later and again for a third and final time after a further fortnight. Either of the dosage schemes will restrain fungation and reduce discharge; if the full dose can be given, the ulceration will usually heal. As the fields of irradiation are aimed tangentially and do not penetrate the body, treatment will not be associated with general systemic symptoms. The only disturbance to the patient will be that with full dosage, the skin of the breast will become mildly erythematous and the nipple temporarily tender.

Other tumours fungating on to the surface of the body may warrant irradiation in an attempt to reduce a profuse discharge. A very elderly lady at St Christopher's Hospice had a huge fungating tumour on the anterior abdominal wall from a primary carcinoma of the gall-bladder. This tumour was expected to be of only moderate radiosensitivity and, as it had been previously irradiated, further treatment was associated with a risk of producing a fistula. But she had no distant metastases and as the only symptom which was keeping her in hospital was a profuse discharge (such that she was unable to stand without soaking her clothing) it seemed justifiable to risk retreatment. A maximum surface dose to the tumour of 1500 rads in three doses was sufficient to control the discharge and allow her to return home, and treatment was safely repeated on two occasions within 6 months before she died.

Patients with advanced rectal carcinoma whose obstructive symptoms have been relieved by a palliative colostomy sometimes live many months with distressing residual symptoms. Severe perineal pain or profuse rectal discharge of mucus from an unremoved primary tumour are difficult to control but a short course of palliative irradiation aimed at the tumour is worth considering as these patients have often had no previous radiotherapy (see Chapter 6).

Control of cough and dyspnoea

Cough and dyspnoea from an advanced primary bronchial carcinoma can often be relieved or improved by a course of palliative radiotherapy. A history of a previous course of palliative irradiation, especially if it has been temporarily successful, does not preclude a second course. Using a simple technique involving a pair of parallel opposed fields, a maximum tumour dose of 2500 rads can be delivered to the primary tumour and mediastinal nodes in six treatments over a period of 3 weeks.

Palliative irradiation of lung metastases should not be considered unless the metastases are from highly radiosensitive tumours such as lymphomas, seminomas or nephroblastomas. In these instances part or all of both lungs can be irradiated. It is, however, unwise to exceed a maximum dose to both lungs of 1500 rads in six treatments over 3 weeks because of the risk of producing an acute radiation pneumonitis. The irradiation of less radiosensitive tumours is unlikely to be of value.

Radiation of large lymph node masses

Enlarged metastatic lymph nodes in the mediastinum from a primary bronchial carcinoma or from a malignant lymphoma may cause the syndrome of
superior vena caval obstruction. The resultant dyspnoea and congestion are
particularly distressing. Occasionally these symptoms can be relieved by therapy with corticosteroids, but not infrequently a course of concurrent radiotherapy similar to that recommended for the relief of cough and dyspnoea will be
of greater value. It is usually wise to irradiate these patients as in-patients
rather than by out-patient visits. Very occasionally the first treatment may be
associated with an exacerbation of the symptoms, although this appears to be
less common than reported in the literature.

It may also be of value to irradiate radiosensitive tumours or nodal metastases
if they are causing obstructive symptoms such as dysphagia in the last few
weeks of life. A primary carcinoma of the oesophagus is not a particularly
radiosensitive tumour but an anaplastic carcinoma of the thyroid causing
dysphagia often responds.

Intra-abdominal metastases from a seminoma of the testis or a dysgerminoma
of the ovary are very radiosensitive and even if large are worth irradiating.

Symptoms unlikely to be helped by radiotherapy

In general, the irradiation of extensive intra-abdominal carcinomatosis from a
carcinoma of the gut or ovary is unrewarding. Even at palliative dosage, such
a course of treatment is often associated with distressing nausea, vomiting and
diarrhoea. In these circumstances well chosen chemotherapy may be preferable or it may be a time to withhold active treatment.

Radiotherapy is rarely, if ever, helpful in the control of pleural effusion or
ascites. In the past, the instillation of radioactive gold was used, but more
recently the instillation of a cytotoxic chemotherapy agent, such as thiotepa,
has been found equally effective and much safer to use.

Side-effects of radiotherapy

The aim of palliative radiotherapy is to relieve symptoms with the lowest
possible dose in the fewest possible treatments. Side-effects at the level of
dosage described in this chapter are unlikely to be severe except for the inevitable nausea produced by fields directed at the epigastrium.

Irradiation of fungating tumours on the surface of the body where a maximum dose falls on the skin may be associated with a temporarily uncomfortable erythema. This can be reduced to a minimum by keeping the irradiated
skin dry and avoiding the application of lotions, ointments or adhesives containing metal salts, such as zinc. Fungating tumours have to be kept clean and
free from infection (see Chapter 6) but unnecessary washing should be avoided
when possible. However, when irradiating the perineum the benefits of brief
bathing far outweigh those of the avoidance of washing.

Mucosal reactions in the mouth and oesophagus are unusual at palliative
dosage but as irradiation predisposes to mucosal infection with Monilia, it is
wise to accompany irradiation with a prophylactic course of an antimonilial

drug such as amphotericin lozenges (10 mg four times daily). Irradiation of the mouth reduces the secretion of saliva and tends to dry the mouth. If food collects in the sulcus and the lips become dry and cracked, advice on oral hygiene can prevent a great deal of suffering.

Temporary diarrhoea may follow palliative irradiation of the pelvis but it should only be moderate at the doses recommended. Kaolin and morphine mixture (10 ml three to six times daily) and codeine phosphate tablets (15–30 mg three times daily) are the most commonly prescribed remedies and, with adequate fluid replacement, should control this side-effect. The mucosa of the bladder is more resistant to irradiation and a course of palliative radiotherapy aimed at controlling haematuria is unlikely to cause troublesome bladder symptoms. Persistent dysuria and frequency are more likely to be due to the effects of the tumour itself.

Prochloperazine (5–10 mg three times daily) is probably the most useful drug to control radiation-induced nausea and vomiting, and a liberal intake of glucose fluids also helps.

It must, however, be stressed that it is unusual to see side-effects from the type of palliative irradiation that has been described for use in the last few months of life. These patients are already ill and it is important not to confuse the progressive symptoms of disease with the symptoms produced by radiotherapy. However, on occasion, patients may be comforted by the erroneous belief that their symptoms are due to a recent course of radiotherapy and this need not disturb a radiotherapist. What matters is the result of good care.

The care of a patient who is terminally ill, and of his family, is at its best when a team of experts work together. It is possible for the surgeon, the radio-therapist and the chemotherapist to deprive a patient of his final dignity but it is also possible that working skilfully together they can contribute to his comfort.

8

Palliation by Cytotoxic Chemotherapy and Hormone Therapy

Thelma D. Bates and Thérèse Vanier

The use of cytotoxic chemotherapy and hormone therapy, though rarely curative, belongs primarily in the active phase of treatment of malignant disease. Because most of the cytotoxic drugs and some of the hormones have unpleasant side-effects, and as a response to treatment may be delayed for several weeks, their use in the terminal stages of malignant disease is very limited. However, although the palliative value of such treatment is not as predictable as that of radiotherapy, a successful response to these drugs is more likely to be associated with a prolongation of life. As with all other modalities of treatment, it is the quality of this life which is important.

At the moment, there are approximately 35 clinically useful cytotoxic drugs. None of them specifically damages malignant cells, and most act by interfering with cell division and cause a variable degree of damage to normal as well as to malignant cells. This leads to unwanted side-effects such as bone marrow depression and gastrointestinal disturbances, thus limiting their use.

Each of the cytotoxic drugs is of value in the treatment of several different tumours, and a higher response rate may often be obtained if several drugs are combined. The most successful combinations in use comprise three or four drugs which are individually effective against the tumour, each having a different mode of action and toxic side-effects which do not overlap. Cytotoxic drugs are also best given intermittently rather than continuously. This helps to avoid the development of drug resistance and immunosuppression which may be important if the expectation of life is to be increased.

Cytotoxic chemotherapy has to be modified and simplified for use in the terminally ill when the emphasis is on symptom control. Unpleasant side-effects, which may be acceptable in the earlier phases of the disease, are no longer justified at this stage. Whenever possible, the drugs used should be effective by mouth, should require the minimum of specialist supervision and monitoring, and should have minimal, controllable side-effects. The drugs chlorambucil and cyclophosphamide satisfy these criteria. Both can be given by mouth and are effective against several solid tumours, including carcinomas of the ovary and breast, as well as lymphomas. When drugs have to be given intravenously, regimens should be simple and the frequency of injections kept to a minimum. Dosage also may have to be modified in order to balance the likely benefit to the patient against the side-effects.

Carcinomas of the breast, endometrium and prostate may respond to sex hormone therapy. By the time these patients reach the terminal stages of their disease, most will have exhausted this form of therapy; but, if not, hormone therapy can be considered. Hormones have several advantages over cytotoxic drugs. They have fewer side-effects, can usually be given by mouth and need less specialist supervision and monitoring. The main disadvantage of both sex hormones and cytotoxic agents in terminal cancer is that a response to treatment often takes 4–6 weeks to become apparent.

Prednisone and dexamethasone play an important role in terminal care as they act quickly and help to relieve a variety of symptoms (Chapters 5 and 6). When given with cytotoxic drugs, they are alleged to give some marrow protection and to reduce nausea.

In general, a pre-existing course of cytotoxic drugs or hormones is stopped in these patients when the disease process shows no sign of control despite adequate duration and level of dosage. There may, however, be a place for continuing low dosage of these agents, even when there is little chance of affecting the disease process, if the patient believes they are beneficial. It is not always easy to know whether the drug is responsible for an apparently static condition. Drugs may be inappropriate at one moment but if the patient's general condition improves and a longer prognosis is evident, they should be considered.

Experience at St Christopher's Hospice over a two-year period is shown in Tables 8.1 and 8.2. In the case of most patients referred to this specialist unit for terminal care, a decision will already have been reached that cytotoxic or hormone treatment is no longer appropriate. In a small number of cases, referral is made primarily for pain or other symptom control but with the option of continuing more aggressive treatment if this is considered appropriate. Stopping what is looked upon as active therapy will be much less traumatic if symptom control has been seen by patient and doctor as of major importance throughout treatment. The figures given for continuing or starting hormone treatment (7 per cent of total admissions) and cytotoxic treatment (3 per cent of total admissions) reflect the general principles underlying the use of these drugs at the present time, as does the breakdown of figures relating to primary sites. We submit that survival figures from St Christopher's Hospice reflect not so much the effect of these drugs as the stage at which patients are transferred to its care.

Breast carcinoma

Patients with breast carcinoma often respond to cytotoxic drugs or to hormones. The choice of treatment will be dictated by the patient's previous response to treatment, her general condition and the estimated possible survival. Cytotoxic drugs may show their earliest effects within 2 or 3 weeks but with hormones one usually has to wait for 4–6 weeks. There is often a place for giving both together.

Single cytotoxic agents

Although single agents are not as effective as multiple drug regimens, they have an important role in the terminally ill because they are often less toxic

Table 8.1   Analysis of patients receiving cytotoxic drugs at St Christopher's Hospice, 1.9.74–31.8.76

Primary site of tumour	Number	% total admissions	Number given cytotoxic drugs	% for tumours at this site	Continued	Started
Breast	192	17	13	6·8	7	6
Gastrointestinal	271	24	9	3	2	7
Bronchus	271	24	3	1	2	1
Ovary	45	4	7	16	3	4
Melanoma	15	1·3	3	20	3	0
Head and neck	40	3·5	1	2·5	0	1
Central nervous system	48	4·2	1	2	1	0
Other	248	22	0	0	0	0
Total	1130	100	37	3·3	18	19

Survival in days	Mean	Median
Treated with cytotoxics	73	42
Drug(s) started	66	49
Drug(s) continued	40	25
(All admissions (1975)*	24	12)

Alive at the end of the study
3 with breast carcinoma (120, 400 and 402 days) (1 received hormones concurrently and 1 received hormones after failure of cytotoxics)

* There has been little change in these figures over the past few years.

Table 8.2   Analysis of patients receiving sex hormones at St Christopher's Hospice, 1.9.74–31.8.76

Primary site of tumour	Number	% total admissions	Number given sex hormones	% for tumours at this site	Continued	Started
Breast	192	17	56	29	46	10*
Prostate	23	2	20	87	20	0
Cervix	28	2·5	1	3·6	1	0
Kidney	17	1·5	3	18	3	0
Endometrium	17	1·5	1	6	1	0
Other	853	75·5	0	0	0	0
Total	1130	100	81	7	71	10

*Includes change of hormone in 2 patients.

Survival in days	Mean	Median
Treated with hormones	51	29
Drug(s) started	217	70
Drug(s) continued	32	27
(All admissions (1975)	24	12)

Alive at the end of the study
1 with carcinoma prostate (450 days)
3 with carcinoma breast (402,† 120,† 60 days)

† Also received cytotoxics.

and simpler to administer. Probably the most useful is cyclophosphamide, which can be expected to cause a temporary but worthwhile response in one-third of cases. It can be given by mouth at a dose of 100 mg daily. Nausea, bone marrow depression and alopecia at this dosage are rare and, if the drug is taken in the morning with plenty of fluids throughout the day, bladder irritation can be avoided. Although intravenous adriamycin is the most effective single agent for breast cancer, a high incidence of alopecia makes it unsuitable for these patients. Intravenous 5-fluorouracil 500 mg at weekly intervals is a well tolerated alternative to oral cyclophosphamide.

Mrs S., aged 76, was admitted mainly for social reasons, with a local recurrence and multiple skin deposits. During the year she lived at St Christopher's she received three courses of oral cyclophosphamide (100 mg daily for 6, 9 and 4 weeks). The first two courses were followed by complete disappearance of the lesions. Despite deterioration in her general condition she was sufficiently troubled by the local recurrence on the chest wall to justify a trial of 5-fluorouracil after the third course of cyclophosphamide was ineffective. She received three weekly injections of 500 mg but the drug was of no avail and she died 3 weeks later.

Mrs P., aged 65, was referred for terminal care with local recurrence, involvement of the opposite breast and secondaries in bone, liver, skin and lymph nodes. Her general condition was remarkably good and she was up and dressed for most of the day shortly after admission. She was started on a combination of cyclophosphamide 100 mg daily and tamoxifen 20 mg twice daily, which caused rapid regression of node and skin secondaries. She is at home, leading a fairly active life 4 months after starting treatment.

Multiple cytotoxic agents

More aggressive cytotoxic therapy may occasionally be justified in patients with gross fungating tumours, especially those which have presented late in the course of the disease. The following intravenous quadruple regimen can be given to out-patients:

Day 1		Day 8	
Cyclophosphamide	500 mg	Cyclophosphamide	500 mg
Vincristine	1 mg	Vincristine	1 mg
5-Fluorouracil	750 mg	Methotrexate	50 mg

Each drug is injected singly into a butterfly needle and washed through with saline. Injections are given on two days a week apart, and repeated after three clear weeks. Patients usually complain of nausea on the day of injection and approximately half will develop alopecia. Full peripheral blood counts must be done before each course of injections. A worthwhile response lasting several months can be expected in 50–60 per cent of patients and improvement is usually apparent in the responders within a month.

Mrs R., aged 67, had been given oestrogen therapy for 4 months before referral but without any benefit. Her general condition was remarkably good despite a gross fungating lesion and leukoerythroblastic anaemia. Because these were causing her dominant symptoms she was transfused with 2 pints blood and treated for 15 months with a quadruple chemotherapy regimen (cyclophosphamide 300 mg, vincristine 1 mg, 5-

fluorouracil 500 mg on day 1, and cyclophosphamide 300 mg, vincristine 1 mg and methotrexate 50 mg on day 8, together with 10 mg metoclopramide (Maxolon) i.v. on each occasion), which produced no significant side-effects. The primary lesion dried up and shrunk considerably and the post transfusion haemoglobin level of 8 g per cent rose spontaneously to 12 g per cent. When she relapsed, tamoxifen 20 mg twice daily was substituted, and at the time of writing she is again in remission and at home.

Hormone therapy

The most useful hormone for the terminally ill is tamoxifen. This anti-oestrogen may benefit both pre- and postmenopausal patients and also those patients who have failed to respond to other hormones. It is given by mouth at a dose of 20 mg twice daily and is remarkably non-toxic. This is the best sex hormone to combine with cytotoxic therapy and is recommended for use with oral cyclophosphamide.

Premarin, a natural oestrogen, is less likely to cause nausea than stilboestrol. A dose of 1·25 mg is equivalent to stilboestrol 5 mg and may be of value in elderly patients with a longer prognosis even if they have failed to respond to other hormones.

Of the androgens, fluoxymesterone is the least virilizing oral preparation. A dose of 10 mg thrice daily can be given to both pre- and postmenopausal patients especially those with skeletal metastases.

Mrs W., aged 63, presented for terminal care with bilateral breast involvement and pleural effusion. She failed to respond to quadruple chemotherapy but responded to tamoxifen 10 mg twice daily and continues to live a fairly normal life 18 months later.

Mrs P., aged 50, was admitted with a 3-year history of breast carcinoma and bone metastases. She had been previously treated with androgens and recently had sustained pathological fractures of both femoral necks—one of which had been pinned. She was thought to be terminally ill and in need of pain control. After this was achieved it became evident that she was well enough to return home, albeit in a wheelchair. Tamoxifen 20 mg twice daily was started in the hope of holding up the progress of the disease and, if possible, preventing further pathological fractures. Five months later she remains fairly well at home and the dose of diamorphine required for pain control has been reduced from 40 mg orally 4-hourly to 30 mg.

Ovarian carcinoma

This tumour does not respond to hormone therapy and, in most patients seen in the terminal stage, cytotoxic drugs will already have been used. If not, they should be considered especially when recurrent ascites requires frequent tapping. The most useful and least toxic drug for these patients is chlorambucil given in an initial dose of 5 mg twice daily. Full blood counts will be necessary at monthly intervals but at this dose level the drug has few side-effects. Less effective alternatives are cyclophosphamide tablets 100 mg daily, treosulphan tablets 250 mg thrice daily or the intraperitoneal instillation of thiotepa 60 mg. Of the drugs not yet available for general use, cis-platinum, which is given intravenously, looks the most promising.

Miss M., aged 70, had refused laparotomy after presenting with severe ascites. Cytology of the ascitic fluid had been unhelpful but there was a large mass arising from the pelvis and disseminating ovarian carcinoma was considered the most likely diagnosis. At first, tapping of 10–15 litres was required monthly to keep her comfortable. Chlorambucil and cyclophosphamide were then used sequentially (chlorambucil 5 mg daily for 2 months, then alternating 2-week periods on 10 mg daily for 5 months; cyclophosphamide 100 mg daily for 3 months and then 50 mg daily for 10 months) and only one further paracentesis was required over the following 18 months despite a gradual increase in the size of the abdominal mass.

Mrs P., aged 68, was found at laparotomy to have an ovarian carcinoma with pelvic and peritoneal spread. Radiotherapy had been started at the referring hospital but was discontinued because of a deterioration in her general condition. She improved to such an extent following admission for terminal care that chlorambucil 10 mg daily was started. She was discharged under the care of her general practitioner and lived a comparatively normal life for 13 months before dying at home.

Endometrial carcinoma

This tumour occasionally responds to progestogens but rarely to cytotoxic drugs. When progestogens have not been used previously they can be tried in the terminally ill; none of these agents has unpleasant side-effects. The most useful drug is medroxyprogesterone acetate (Provera), which can be given by mouth at a dose of 100 mg twice daily. An alternative is a weekly intramuscular injection of gestronol heyanoate (Depostat) 200 mg.

Cervical carcinoma

The rare adenocarcinomas of the cervix may respond to progestogens in a similar way to endometrial adenocarcinoma but the common squamous cell carcinoma of the cervix does not respond to hormones. The most useful cytotoxic agents are adriamycin and methotrexate, but as both are highly toxic drugs they cannot be recommended for the terminally ill. If the expectation of life is somewhat greater, intravenous adriamycin 50 mg and methotrexate 20 mg on day 1 and methotrexate 20 mg on day 8 may temporarily relieve pelvic pain and bleeding.

Gastrointestinal carcinoma

The long-term results of cytotoxic therapy in this form of cancer are not encouraging. Less than 10 per cent of admissions to St Christopher's Hospice with this type of primary will have been given such treatment.

Patients with pelvic spread due to carcinoma of the rectum may live a long time and pain control may be particularly difficult. Radiotherapy remains the best palliative adjuvant to analgesics, but 5-fluorouracil may be useful if radiotherapy is contraindicated.

Mrs R., aged 41, presented with gross pelvic invasion, including involvement of the vaginal vault. Pain was controlled with oral diamorphine but troublesome vaginal bleeding and discharge persisted when an effective pain control regimen allowed her to return home to care for a young family. Intravenous 5-fluorouracil was given, 500 mg weekly and then fortnightly over a period of 3 months, and these symptoms cleared during this time. Subsequently, increase in pain, liver involvement and general deterioration necessitated readmission and she died 3 weeks later.

Mrs Y., aged 53, was referred because of gross pelvic spread, severe pain, vaginal discharge and bleeding. Two courses of quadruple chemotherapy at the referring hospital had made her feel very ill. When pain had been relieved with oral diamorphine, intravenous 5-fluorouracil 500 mg weekly and later fortnightly controlled the vaginal symptoms for several months. This allowed her to be at home for 7 out of the 11 months she lived after referral for terminal care.

Not surprisingly, 5-fluorouracil is largely ineffective in controlling pain when used by itself in gastrointestinal cancer, but on rare occasions has proved helpful for pain due to carcinoma of the head of the pancreas.

Prostatic carcinoma

Most patients with prostatic carcinoma will be receiving hormone treatment, commonly stilboestrol (5–25 mg three times daily). This is usually continued into the terminal phase but the dosage may be reduced if the patient is vomiting or nauseated, or shows signs of fluid retention. A decision to start hormone treatment at this time is rare (see Table 8.2).

Bronchial carcinoma

Because of its poor response to cytotoxic drugs, no more than 5 per cent of lung cancer patients referred to St Christopher's have been treated in this way except for small cell anaplastic ('oat cell') carcinomas. It is important to establish the exact histology since single agents such as cyclophosphamide may produce a remission of symptoms even if this is short-lived.

In the main, symptoms due to bronchial carcinoma are better controlled by radiotherapy or nerve block in conjunction with appropriate medication. In our opinion, tapping pleural effusion in the terminal stages either for fluid removal or instillation of a cytotoxic is rarely helpful as reaccumulation is rapid to the previous level. Dyspnoea is best controlled by small doses of morphine or diamorphine (Chapter 6).

Head and neck carcinoma

Occasionally, patients with severe pain due to advanced squamous cell carcinoma in the head and neck can be helped temporarily by a course of intramuscular bleomycin. A dose of 15 mg twice weekly for 3–4 weeks is recommended for patients who have not had this cytotoxic drug previously. Side-effects will include nausea and fever; pulmonary fibrosis can be avoided if the total dose from all courses does not exceed 300 mg.

Lymphoproliferative disorders and leukaemias

Patients with these malignancies come into a special category in relation to cytotoxic agents. They will all have been treated with such drugs and also usually with blood and blood products. By the time they are terminally ill such treatment has become a way of life. This may make the decision to stop such treatment more difficult, but the change in emphasis will be easier if attention to symptom control is given greater prominence as the disease progresses.

Summary

When patients enter what is thought to be the terminal stages of malignant disease, the emphasis in treatment is on the control of distressing symptoms. On rare occasions cytotoxic drugs and hormones can be used to relieve these symptoms and in doing so they may sometimes prolong life. As long as accurate prognosis remains difficult, these agents will continue to be useful.

9

The Place of Surgery in Terminal Care

Michael R. Williams

While there is still a prospect of cure or long-term control of disease, one can reasonably demand a great deal of patients in terms of pain, discomfort and time. Extensive ablations of tumour masses, amputations of limbs, the cosmetic disfigurement of major dissections of the head and neck—combined if necessary with exacting courses of radiotherapy and cytotoxic drugs—are all worth their while. But once the progress of the disease makes it clear that cure is no longer possible, the emphasis of treatment must be changed to secure the maximum quality of life for the period that remains at the cost of the minimum morbidity. Morbidity includes not only pain and discomfort but also loss of independence and dignity, clouding of consciousness and time spent in hospital. For those who have a home to go to, every day spent in even the best hospital is a day wasted which can be ill-afforded when life is limited.

There are some symptoms which no patient should suffer for long:

> Intestinal colic;
> Protracted vomiting;
> Inability to swallow one's own saliva.

To which I would add

> The stench of secondarily infected fungating lesions;
> The intractable itch of unrelieved obstructive jaundice;
> Faecal or urinary incontinence;
> The throbbing pain of pus under tension.

When these symptoms arise they must be controlled. On occasion radiotherapy and cytotoxic drugs may make a considerable contribution to palliation of the patient's symptoms (see Chapters 7 and 8). Failing that, control can almost always be achieved by adequate drug therapy which (if necessary) can be justifiably pushed to the point of shortening life; even without doing this, the dosage necessary to secure control may depress the level of awareness and deprive the patient of his independence and ability to exist outside an institution.

It may be possible, however, to provide relief by surgery at the cost of a lesser morbidity, in which case it is essential to count the cost. Apart from minor procedures such as draining abscesses which are justifiable in the last days, my own rule of thumb is that one week spent in a surgical ward is justifiable if there is a prospect of three months' useful life at home, two weeks for six months' respite, while three weeks in hospital is justified for a year of worthwhile survival.

When presented with a patient with incurable malignant disease one should assess the present symptoms and signs and, in the light of the likely natural history of the disease, attempt to predict symptoms which may occur as the condition progresses and which are likely to prove troublesome and unacceptable. One then tries to devise some programme which will relieve the former and obviate the latter. The essence of effective terminal care is long-term planning so that the problems in the last days are manageable. Such planning implies working out an individual programme for each problem, using a common set of principles.

Take, for example, a patient with carcinoma of the rectum. The associated symptoms may be considered in two main groups: those due to the presence of the tumour itself and those due to the narrowing of the lumen of the bowel. (A third group of symptoms, due to the general systemic effects of advanced malignant disease, are described in Chapters 2 and 3.) The tumour will cause by its presence increased mucus secretion, rectal bleeding and tenesmus. Fungating lesions are likely to become infected, with development of local abscesses and fistulae. The tumour may spread locally and involve adjacent tissues such as other pelvic viscera, the sacral plexus or anal skin, and it may cause venous obstruction with oedema of the legs. If the tumour obstructs the lumen of the bowel the patient will develop colic, frequent and uncontrollable diarrhoea or incontinence and, finally, as the obstruction progresses, abdominal distension and vomiting.

A colostomy will relieve only the obstructive symptoms. Whenever possible, it is more satisfactory to remove the primary lesion and at least reduce the chances of local recurrence during the likely period of survival. If a patient at laparotomy is found to have a moderate amount of metastatic disease in his liver and he is likely to live a year or more, he will be best served by an abdominoperineal resection: this procedure will remove his primary tumour and reduce the risk of local recurrence at the cost of three weeks or a little less in hospital. With extensive hepatic metastases and a shorter prognosis of only six months or so, this approach would be inappropriate. It may, however, be possible to mobilize the tumour sufficiently to resect it and close the stump of the rectum below (Hartmann's operation), bringing out a terminal colostomy which must be carefully sutured to the skin with silk sutures to secure primary mucocutaneous healing. The patient can then begin to care for his colostomy without delay and, with no perineal wound to heal, he can be home in ten days.

If the primary tumour cannot be removed, a colostomy should be performed only if the patient has obstructive symptoms. In their absence a colostomy is only an added burden. With a simple laparotomy and closure, the patient will be able to return to his family in a few days. If he develops colic later, a colostomy is a simple matter; but it may never prove necessary and a colostomy as such will do nothing to prevent the symptoms produced by the tumour itself.

If the patient has obstructive symptoms and a colostomy is performed, the bowel should always be divided and the proximal end carefully sutured to the skin with interrupted silk stitches to secure primary mucocutaneous healing with minimal reaction. The patient can then start to care for his own colostomy as soon as it works. In my view there is no place in palliative surgery for the cumbersome loop colostomy which requires the assistance of nurses until it shrinks down. The distal end is best closed and dropped back into the abdomen. It never seems to give trouble and, by not bringing it out on the abdominal wall, one reduces the risk of a local metastatic deposit in the skin. The colostomy should be sited so that the patient can reach it easily himself even though the abdomen may subsequently become distended with a large liver or ascites. Continuing independence is more important than cosmetic appearance.

Using the same principles and lines of thought, a suitable plan can be produced for the management of incurable malignant disease at any site using surgery, radiotherapy, cytotoxic drugs and simple medicament as indicated. Each programme must be planned on an individual basis, treating the patient in the context of his disease rather than the disease itself.

In general, removal of the primary tumour wherever possible is desirable in any lesion which is likely to fungate either on the surface of the skin or in the lumen of the bowel. This is particularly important with carcinoma of the breast where an offensive ulcerated mass can readily be removed and primary healing at least temporarily secured by some form of local mastectomy; this may well be accompanied by hormonal therapy in suitable cases, either by drugs or by ablative surgery.

The surgeon should resist the temptation to refer such patients for radio-therapy merely as a method of disposal. Radiotherapy should be advised only after careful discussion with the other colleagues in the team, taking into account the possible advantages and disadvantages for that particular patient.

Even in the last stages, it is often worthwhile to excise particularly trouble-some skin metastases, which can often be done under local anaesthesia.

To revert to the gastrointestinal tract. Patients with intestinocutaneous fistulae may have pain from inadequate drainage and secondary abscesses which are frequently subcutaneous, lying superficial to the muscles. Laying the fistulae widely open and saucerizing the abscesses will relieve the pain instantly and make the lesions easier to dress by the district nurse at home.

If persistent colic is a problem, not controlled by danthron with poloxamer (Dorbanex) and enemas, and if there appear to be some months of useful life left, a fistula should be established proximal to the obstruction—either a colostomy or even an ileostomy. It is a mistake to think that the latter is particularly troublesome to the patient with modern appliances. Mucocutaneous suture should always be done and training in the management of the stoma must be begun at once.

If it is clear at laparotomy that there are multiple obstructed loops of bowel secondary to numerous peritoneal seedlings on the serosal surfaces (as it is often the case in disseminating carcinomas of the ovary), no attempt should be made to separate these or perform several side-to-side anastomoses for fear of producing multiple fistulae. It is wiser to close the abdomen and control the symptoms with adequate analgesia. The same is true of obstruction in the last stages of the disease, when the patient is unlikely to have long enough to enjoy the relief he has earned through the discomforts and stress of the operation.

Each case must be considered on its merits, taking into account not only the disease and the stage it has reached but also the patient's particular problems and aspirations. A woman with two boys at boarding school was dying from recurrent carcinoma of the cervix causing colonic obstruction. The ureters were also involved and her blood urea was raised, but her principal problem was uncontrollable diarrhoea which kept her house-bound. A terminal colostomy with mucocutaneous suture was performed in the third week of July and she was out of hospital in seven days looking after her own colostomy. She was able to accompany the boys on various expeditions, visiting the theatre twice and going to restaurants and museums throughout the summer holidays. She died of uraemia a few days after the beginning of term. In spite of the shortness of the respite this was worth her while.

Fungating lymph node metastases in the neck, axilla and groin present particular problems. In advanced cases it is rarely possible to achieve surgical clearance. Radiotherapy and cytotoxic drugs may help to control pain, but are unlikely to secure healing. Secondary infection of surrounding normal tissues can be controlled by courses of systemic antibiotics but it is impossible to sterilize the fungating lesion. The local management of fungating tumours is dealt with in Chapter 6.

Death in such cases may well be from secondary haemorrhage (see Chapter 2). If haemorrhage occurs, there is no place for resuscitation and transfusion: narcotic drugs in adequate dosage, to which hyoscine 0·4 mg can usefully be added, must be instantly available. Normally there is a small warning bleed, before the final fatal haemorrhage. This is not an indication to isolate the patient behind screens, but instead he should be encouraged to pursue his normal activities. It is, however, kind to arrange for the traditional red blanket to be draped about him to lessen the distress of any onlookers if a large bleed ensues.

In inoperable carcinoma of the oesophagus and cardia the great problem is that the patient will finally be unable to swallow his own saliva. Every effort must be made to enable him to do this and it is justifiable to incur very considerable risks to achieve it. I find a Mousseau–Barbin tube the best method, but it is essential to trim off the green rim before inserting it (if this is not done the orifice of the tube tends to crinkle up when it is in position and obstruct the lumen). If the tube becomes blocked with food, fizzy drinks or soda water will frequently clear it. On no account should a gastrostomy be established in these patients or they will be kept alive to die of drowning in their own spittle.

In obstructive jaundice, as opposed to the terminal jaundice due to intrahepatic metastases, patients are frequently depressed and much troubled by an intolerable itch; this can be dramatically relieved by free drainage of the bile. In incurable carcinoma of the head of the pancreas, a choledochoduodenostomy with a wide anastomosis is a satisfying procedure because it leaves so little dead space and, consequently, a low risk of cholangitis. Failing this, a cholecystojejunostomy or even an external biliary fistula via a T tube will secure relief. If the obstruction is higher up the biliary system, due either to a carcinoma of the bile duct or external pressure on the duct from enlarged lymph nodes in the porta hepatis, it is sometimes possible to insert a stiff polythene tube up the opened duct through the obstruction, tapping the dilated system above. The tube should be fixed in position with a thread stitch and the common duct closed. The tube may remain patent for some months.

Apart from such specific considerations, there are various points which a surgeon as a member of the team caring for the incurable patient must continually bear in mind.

Urinary and faecal incontinence is very distressing to the patients and their attendants and may be kept hidden from the doctor unless specifically asked for. It is due to overflow until proved otherwise. A urethral catheter, either intermittently released or with free drainage into a bag, can transform the situation. The catheter should be on the small side to prevent irritation of the urethra and, in the male, it is often more satisfactory to use a fine suprapubic catheter such as a Riches which can be inserted blind under local anaesthetic and does not require such frequent changing. The use of antibiotics in catheterized patients is discussed in Chapter 6.

Most analgesics are constipating, and faecal impaction is common. As well as uncontrolled diarrhoea, it may cause considerable perineal discomfort. Once faecal impaction has occurred it is advisable to do a manual removal rather than attempt multiple enemas which are often unrewarding and always exhausting. It is essential to examine the rectum daily for some days afterwards. Reimpaction may occur as further faeces come down from the rest of the colon.

Perineal abscesses, whether secondary to fistulae or arising *de novo*, are frequently overlooked and should be searched for when doing the routine rectal examination to exclude faecal impaction. In the terminally ill, abscesses can arise very insidiously and the site of new pain must always be examined carefully to make sure it is not due to an abscess rather than neural involvement by neoplastic disease. Such discomfort can be relieved by simple drainage of the abscess.

Pus may form under tension beneath a slough of dead tissue in a pressure sore on the buttocks, heels or elbows. Excision of the slough, which does not require an anaesthetic and is painless, will give relief.

Finally, it is a mistake to think of malignant disease as a steadily and relentlessly progressive process. Periods of stabilization between the host and the tumour may occur, either spontaneously or as a result of treatment; occasionally, regression to a dramatic extent may occur. One must be constantly on the lookout for such a fortunate, if unusual, event. The patient should then be reassessed and may well be put back in the category mentioned in the first paragraph where more active therapy such as 'second looks' or active treatment of comparatively minor disabilities may well be appropriate.

To sum up: the surgeon has frequently been involved in the care of the patient in happier days. Once it is clear that the disease is incurable, careful planning and foresight will help to make the last months and weeks as comfortable and valuable to the patient as possible. Even during the last weeks the surgeon may well have something to contribute, and careful reassessment of the patient's problems to see what can be offered is well worthwhile. The surgeon's continuing interest will be a boost to the patient's morale.

10

In-patient Management of Advanced Malignant Disease

T. S. West

Editorial note

J. Englebert Dunphy, in a compelling lecture on Caring for the Patient with Cancer (1976), refers to his experience 30 years ago in the wards of the Home of the Holy Ghost, Cambridge, Massachusetts, and to the superb nursing care he found there. At the end of this most important paper he calls on doctors to look at the spirit which still permeates that and similar homes or hospices.

Those who are concerned with the management of terminal disease today (not only with patients who are dying of cancer), can learn from the experience of the past. Much of it has been in general or cancer hospitals and many of the papers quoted from which we have all been learning came from these sources. From the end of the nineteenth century there have been special homes or hospices on both sides of the Atlantic, in Australia and elsewhere, derived in their turn from the mediaeval resting places for travellers or pilgrims, the deaconess hospitals of Europe and from the work of the Irish Sisters of Charity. Many of them are still active, continuing the work for which they were founded but gradually becoming involved with the new potentials in terminal care.* We note that hospitals founded at that time for the chronic sick have more often turned to acute medicine as new treatments have become available to their patients and only a few of these still include the dying as a special concern.

It seems that at the end of the nineteenth century patients were often neglected or ostracized. It was seeing their desperation as they were banished to the almshouse on Welfare Island, New York, and to the Poor Law Institutions of London that impelled Rose Hawthorne and Dr Howard Barrett to begin their work at St Rose's Home and St Luke's Hospital. Hospices were needed because patients frequently had too *little* treatment, whereas today some of the 'hospice movement' in the United States is stimulated by what is seen as too *much*, and often inappropriate, treatment. 'Medical advances have lengthened for many people the time between the diagnosis of a fatal malignancy and the patient's death. This has exacerbated the problems of chronic pain, fear, dependency, loss of self-esteem and progressive dehumanization for many persons' (Feifel, 1977). The hopes for success of some of the more recent treatments, even at a late stage of the disease, have made decisions concerning what is appropriate both more pressing and more difficult. Such decisions can be made easier where adequate terminal care is available. New methods of giving such care are developing.

* For example, The Hostel of God, St Luke's Hospice (now Hereford Lodge), St Columba's Hospital, St Joseph's Hospice and, from the 1950s, the Homes of the Marie Curie Memorial Foundation and others in the United Kingdom. In the United States of America, the Homes of the Hawthorne Dominicans, Youville Hospital, Boston (formerly Home of the Holy Ghost), Calvary Hospital and others.

West's chapter presents the care which is offered to these patients in today's 'hospices'—the hospitality and concern for people, individual decisions concerning the treatments discussed (see Chapters 5–9) and the building of the whole ward team which makes this possible.

Nuttall points out the distress, often amounting to despair, which is felt by many nurses who do not find this care being offered to their patients—whatever the reason. Her reference to the discussions developing between the Colleges concerned is a cause for optimism.

Ford's chapter is not an official presentation of the role of the National Health Service in this field but comes from her own experience, not only in the Department of Health and Social Security, but first as a regular medical visitor at St Christopher's Hospice. Like the Editor, she finds a week-end as the only doctor on duty is the best way to study the management of terminal malignant disease and to meet the challenge of interpreting it wherever such patients are to be found.

References and further reading

ABRAMS, R. D. (1974). *Not Alone with Cancer*. Charles C. Thomas; Springfield, Illinois.

DUNPHY, J. E. (1976). Annual discourse—on caring for the patient with cancer. *New England Journal of Medicine* **295**, 313.

FEIFEL, H. (1959). *The Meaning of Death*. McGraw-Hill; New York.

FEIFEL, H. (Ed.) (1977). *Death in Contemporary America*, in New Meanings of Death. McGraw-Hill; New York and Maidenhead.

FULTON, R. (1965, 1976). *Death and Identity*, 1st and 2nd edns. Charles Press; Bowie, Maryland.

GLASER, B. G. and STRAUSS, A. L. (1966). *Awareness of Dying*. Weidenfeld & Nicolson, London.

KUBLER-ROSS, E. (1970). *Death and Dying*. Tavistock Publications; London.

STODDARD, S. (1978). *The Hospice Movement—A Better Way of Caring for the Dying*. Stein and Day, New York.

WEISMAN, A. D. (1972). *Dying and Denying—a psychiatric study of terminality*. Behavioral Publications; New York.

'My Rule is to receive you with hospitality and to let you go in peace.'
From Sayings of the Desert Fathers

The need for admission

Some patients suffering from advanced malignant disease will need admission. However competent the general practitioner, or however willing the family, situations may arise when full-time skilled nursing and medical care will become essential if the patient's symptoms are to be properly controlled (Saunders, 1973).

Admission may be precipitated by any of the following.

1. Inability to control the symptoms of the disease; for example:
   pain;
   restlessness;
   confusion;
   nausea;
   breathlessness;
   incontinence;
   pressure sores.

2. Breakdown in the family; for example:
exhaustion;
lack of sleep;
concurrent illness;
financial worries;
overwhelming anguish, often associated with a facade of deception.
3. Lack of appropriate social services; for example:
inadequate Social Security benefits;
incontinence laundry;
home adaptations or equipment;
night sitters;
home help.

Admission can be postponed by:

1. Ability of the general practitioner and his team to control the symptoms of the disease and the distress of the patient and the family.
2. A close and competent family and/or good neighbours.
3. The strength which can come from sharing the truth.
4. Full social service support.
5. The security which comes from the knowledge that admission to a suitable bed can be arranged without delay should the need arise.

Preparation to admit

Good management of advanced malignant disease will be achieved only if those concerned are trained:

1. To distinguish between what is appropriate and inappropriate treatment at each stage of this patient's illness.
2. To accept the change of direction from cure to care, and its possible reversal.
3. To learn the special medical and nursing skills involved in competent terminal care.

The phrase 'the doctor said there was nothing more he could do', may sometimes represent a patient or family's misunderstanding of a statement made in a limited context. Sometimes it really has been said, yet the combined skills of teams caring for people who are dying consistently refute this conclusion (Saunders, 1975).

Little imagination is needed to picture the usual course such patients will have followed before they are admitted for terminal care. A long series of hopes and disappointments, of various more or less successful treatments and of relating to a host of new medical and nursing faces will have left the patient exhausted, often despairing and sometimes cynical. The first step must be for the staff in the new ward to be interested enough to make the patient feel wanted and welcome as himself rather than for his physical condition, and also confident that they can deal with the factors which have precipitated his admission.

Admission must be efficient, quick and warm. This is no time for a junior clerk to search for a patient's number or for the patient, trolley and family to be left in a cold corridor. A senior person representing the institution should welcome the patient and his family and see them quickly through to the ward where the nurse in charge, having welcomed them herself, should introduce the new arrival to the other patients (and their families) in the bay or ward.

Admission to a specialized unit

Should admission become necessary the general practitioner may have no choice as to where he sends his patient. All the same, neither a geriatric unit nor the busy medical or surgical ward of a general hospital will be appropriate unless the staff of the ward concerned have time and enthusiasm for terminal care.

A specialized unit or hospice dealing mainly with terminal care may be available. Such a place might be thought to engender a death-house image (as indeed could the Palliative Care Unit or the Symptom Control Team—or the screened bed or single room at the end of the ward); but a reputation for nursing care and symptom control will keep ahead of this image and in practice has been shown to challenge the standard of pain control and terminal care in wards or other institutions that it borders (Melzack, 1976).

A specialized unit is directed towards care rather than cure, possesses a corpus of specialized knowledge, and can provide an appropriate setting for the patient and his family as they come to terms with the final stages of a life. Medical and nursing staff who have the confidence of their own experience in controlling the pains of terminal disease and who do not regard death as a final failure, can sit by a patient's bed and listen to him. With appropriate treatment and successful symptom control, barriers of silence (and of chatter) can be lowered (see Chapter 4). In such an atmosphere the visits of the children can take their rightful and important place.

Admission to the ward

Unless the patient is in pain, the first half-hour after admission should be unhurried. During this time the staff will begin to make their own observations of the patient and the family. The ward staff will inform the doctor if the relatives are in a hurry to leave.

If the patient arrives in pain, he should be seen by the doctor as quickly as possible. Sometimes he will not have been given analgesics that morning. Sometimes a long and uncomfortable ambulance journey will have exacerbated his pain and all drugs will have to be written up before the nursing staff is allowed to administer them.

It is sad to receive a desperately ill person who has been packed off in a sitting ambulance, without adequate drugs for a long journey.

Having obtained information from the notes and from the nurses, the doctor makes the patient welcome. He may then interview the family or friends, for often the patient is ill and tired and it is the family who can best and most easily describe the events which have led up to admission. Of course, it may seem right to interview and examine the patient first and sometimes it seems right to interview husband and wife together.

Admitting the family

Every effort should be made to meet the family and to give them time to talk, for there will never be a more crucial time than the day the patient is admitted. The preceding weeks for them may have been as hard or harder than for the patient. If he has come from another hospital the chances are that he is already very ill or that the family, for whatever reason, were unable to have him home. If the patient has come from home the recital of anxiety, pain, soiled linen and sleepless nights, so often told with a minimum of self-pity, can only impress one with the family's love and strength.

Often, however, the family will feel that they have failed the patient by not succeeding in keeping him at home until the end. Part of the doctor's duty is to tell the family that, having seen the patient and having read the doctor's letter, it is obvious that they really have done everything humanly possible and that the patient now needs the full-time nursing care and skills which can be given only with admission.

If the patient has come from home, a lot of the necessary but simple facts can be obtained from the family—'What can he keep down? . . . Is there anything he specially fancies? . . . Alcohol? When did he last get to the bathroom unaided? . . . Is movement a trigger for pain? . . . Is it pain that keeps him awake? . . . Does he sleep during the day? . . . Is he incontinent?'—and here assurance can be given that we are all used to these common problems, and that he need not feel ashamed.

Although some indication of the rate of deterioration may be obtained from the family, in the experience of most doctors an accurate prognosis is impossible. 'Days rather than weeks' or 'weeks rather than months' are probably as far as one should go—with the statement that 'we may be able to tell a little more when we have watched him for a few days'. Sometimes the family are not really asking, 'How long?' but rather, 'What is the end going to be like?' An assurance that symptoms will be controlled and that dying itself will not be distressing (suffocating, choking, painful or isolated) will help to reduce the fears of the unknown which the family may carry as they sit round the patient's bed. Less factual knowledge can also be sought; insight, religious faith and the place truth holds within that family.

Permission to tell the patient 'the truth' as he *wants* and *needs* to know it can almost always be obtained from the family if it is carefully explained to them that this is likely to be a gradual process. The family who has perpetuated the concealment of truth from the patient will need to be assured that they will not be let down, for it may well have been right for them to have carried the burden of knowledge to this point; the patient would have done the same for them. Now they may share—and they often do so.

Often it seems that the family, when first told the diagnosis and prognosis, went into a state of shocked denial on the part of the patient—and of themselves. This may have been appropriate during a period of remission but when the disease begins to progress the family, too often with the connivance of the doctors, continues to deny the patient the truth and lets him walk the lonely path towards realization and dying by himself.

It is wrong and should be unnecessary to tell a patient direct lies. Death from cancer is seldom a sudden catastrophe. If we are sensitive and are travelling with our patient he will be the one who lets us see if and when he is ready to know more about his condition.

By this stage patients who ask for the truth rarely give up when they receive it. Rather, they sum up all that their life has been and, having looked (with their family) at the fact of death, are then better able to live out the time which remains profitably and even happily.

Admitting the patient

The patient may be very ill and tired. His admission need not be long but must appear unhurried. The identification of his main complaints and a general physical examination (which may not have been carried out by a doctor since active treatment was stopped) are probably all that is necessary at this first interview.

The reassurances that we are glad to see him, have taken note of what he complains of and will do something about it and that the bed is his for as long as he needs it are astonishingly therapeutic. Unless it is essential, it is wise not to change medication for the first 24 hours. Previous medication may now become more effective and in any case the first night in a strange place is not the ideal situation to introduce new drugs.

Although the drugs the patient has been taking may no longer be controlling his symptoms, he must be given time to transfer his trust to the new team caring for him. Only then can he be expected to dispense with the old drug regimen on which he has been forced to rely as the only defence against unbearable pain. In practice, by taking the same analgesics he has been given 'on demand' and giving them to him regularly (*before* pain breaks through), previously unrelieved pain can often be controlled (Melzack, 1976). As one patient said to me: 'At St Christopher's you do not pursue the pain, you anticipate it.'

Telling

Quite often, when asked to tell us about their illness, patients will reveal that they are fully aware of their diagnosis; at this first meeting truth can sometimes be brought into the family situation, often with dramatic results.

More often the questions and anxiety which point to a request for the truth come obliquely from the patient and are presented at different times to different members of staff. At St Christopher's Hospice a special pink page is kept in the patient's notes for any member of staff to record conversations that could be of use in the total care of the patient (Fig. 10.1).

On the 21st January I was called to the ward, was shown what had been said, and asked by sister to speak to Mrs D. My subsequent remarks are also shown on Fig. 10.1.

Of course the doctors had seen Mrs D. regularly from the day she was admitted but she had chosen to control the tempo and course of her questions and to direct them to people she felt sure would not push her faster or further than she was ready to go. The simplicity of her questions when they finally reached the doctor are well worth noting . . . she is saying, 'Let me die'—she is not saying, 'Kill me'.

ST.CHRISTOPHER'S HOSPICE

THIS FORM IS FOR THE USE OF ALL NURSING STAFF
FOR NOTING ANY SIGNIFICANT COMMENTS MADE TO THEM BY THE
PATIENT REGARDING HIS/HER ILLNESS AND PROGRESS

PATIENT'S NAME ...MRS. M. D..............

Date

4.1.74 "We're not incurables are we?"
When asked why this statement, patient
replied, "I was just thinking". A.M.M.

7.1.74 Having told me that she wasn't feeling so
well today, she said forcefully, "I'm not
worried about it as I KNOW I'm going
to get better".

20 1 74 Do they know what's wrong with me? Yesterday, I thought I
was dying....... I suppose nobody really knows what's
wrong, do they? M.R.

20.1.74. "I thought this was a convalescent home ...
I wish they would tell me if I've got cancer.....
people do get better from that, don't they?" M.McC.

21.1.74. Gently told that she has got cancer and is dying.
'Will you keep me?' 'Of course'. 'Oh good'.
'Do I have to eat?' 'No' 'Good'. 'Oh good'
'Can I sleep?' 'As much as you like'. 'Oh good'
Seems truly pleased to know. Will share with
family. Not frightened of death. D.G.

Fig. 10.1. Record of conversations with Mrs D.

Who should tell how much and when is a matter for which there is no umbrella answer. We can say that the doctor should never tell a direct lie to a patient, if for no other reason than that the lie will almost certainly be discovered and confidence, not only in the doctor but also in his successors, will be undermined. However, the busy consultant on a teaching round is unlikely to have time to sit down and listen to a patient's hesitant questions. Some consultants make a point of returning alone but it seems reasonable to expect that those who cannot do so should make it clear that responsible members of the team have permission to listen to their patients' questioning and to answer as best they can, and that they will have his support even when things go less than perfectly. Most of us can sympathize with the consultant who said, 'I never tell my patients the truth. I did so once . . .'. But that should not be the end of the story.

To tell a patient he is going 'for convalescence' when in fact he is going to a home for terminal care may get the sending hospital out of an awkward situation; it will almost certainly put the receiving team in a difficult one. Far better to say, 'We are sending you to a place where they have the staff, the skill and the time to give you the care you now need . . .'

The family doctor would seem to be the obvious person to introduce the truth at the appropriate time. Slowness of communication between the hospital and the general practitioner, and then a letter containing a list of findings without any statement about what the family and the patient have been told, do not make his task any easier.

The most important question is not 'What do you tell your patients?' but rather, '*How* do you tell them and what do you let them tell you?' This sounds simple but in practice involves a sensitivity to the questions being asked and to the answers which, at each particular stage in his illness, the patient can accept (Abrams, 1974).

Staff communication

The doctor reports back to the senior nurse and discusses with her his findings, defining the problems and starting to plan for the care of both patient and family. Uncontrolled pain and inadequately shared insight are the two problems which most commonly head the list.

Effective management will depend not only on the skills and knowledge of the medical and nursing staff but also on the speed and ease with which communication can take place between the caring team—which should include the family itself.

Ward reports may be little more than a list of names, procedures, drugs and current practical problems, but there should be a time when the ward sister and her team are able to discuss the problems of particular patients in some depth.

The doctor, doing his round, should first go through the list of patients on the ward with the ward sister, giving her a chance to report to him changes in a patient's condition or anxiety about him or his family. Changes in medication and arrangements, when appropriate, to meet with the family can be planned.

'The doctor's round' itself should normally be done alone. A consultant and his registrar or houseman should go round together sometimes and this can be particularly useful, if they work well as a team, in helping patients and families who are still trying to manipulate the staff in the hope of altering the facts, or who are presenting complicated problems of management—often the physical and emotional are inextricably intertwined. The doctor must give the patient time to talk. Only in this manner will the symptom control discussed in Chapters 5 and 6 be maintained, for 'pain' can be thought of as whatever the patient experiencing it says that it is—not what the doctor thinks that it ought to be, not what the nurses report that it is, not even what the family complain that it is. Very ill patients may take long pauses between perfectly lucid sentences as they look for words and estimate the real interest of their doctor.

Such a careful round should take place at least twice a week; on other days, as long as the nursing staff are experienced, a visit to the patients with specific problems and a few words of greeting to the others in the bay may be all that is necessary.

Although patients who are very ill should be protected from having to meet too many new people, it seems useful if each patient is visited by more than one doctor during the week. Some patients open up to one doctor along a wide but fixed frontier but choose to step over that particular frontier with another doctor with whom they have not developed quite so personal a relationship.

A doctor's visit to a dying person reassures him, the relatives, neighbouring patients and ward staff that 'everything possible is being done'. It is important that after each round the doctor reports back to the nurse in charge of the ward and records any problems or conversations that will be of use to the ward team in the total care of the patient and his family. The whole ward staff must make this journey with the patient and his family and must not stand aloof from his increasing weakness or their exhaustion. They are all involved with the problems of physical distress and may have to support a growing awareness of truth.

Good terminal care requires enough ward staff to sit with patients who are anxious or dying and to spend time with families who are under stress and, later, when they have been bereaved. In most cases temperature, pulse and respiration charts and a number of investigations can usually be dispensed with and the time saved more profitably used. Routine investigations have no place but particular procedures may be indicated in individual patients (Mount, 1976).

When families telephone to enquire about a relative the nursing staff should, if possible, ask the enquirer to wait while they go to see the patient and then report back. The phrase, 'As comfortable as can be expected', has little meaning. Should any member of the family appear to be under dangerous stress, it is the responsibility of the ward to find appropriate support.

Nurses' ward reports and doctors' rounds done in close liaison with the ward sister still leave room for a weekly ward meeting—an opportunity for the exchange of important information. Such a meeting, after the confidence of the staff has been gained, will bring to light anxieties, questions and unrecorded information from the most unlikely sources. This meeting should normally only include staff who work with the patients in that particular ward: doctors and nurses, social workers, physiotherapists, chaplain and others. It must be constructed so that any person present, however junior, feels able to question or contribute. It is a comfort to find that everyone else is also finding a particular patient difficult or that others have noticed with anxiety the strain a particular family is enduring. And it is good to hear of a patient's courage or wit, or of the mutual support families and patients can give the staff as well as each other. The drug management of a patient is sometimes questioned and needs discussion, for although the prescription must finally be written by the doctor, it is the ward staff who will help him to decide what is appropriate treatment and what could be inappropriate and to balance dose levels to individual need.

When lines of communication are properly used the assessment of a patient's pain (be it physical, mental, social or spiritual), concern for the family and signs of strain among the staff should not take too long in coming to light. As a team we gain a broader awareness of unsolved problems and unexpected successes than anyone of us alone can recognize.

The caring team

It is clear that the ward sister rather than the doctor heads the caring team in the ward, unravels the strands and calls in the 'experts'.

The doctor, with his knowledge of appropriately applied pharmacology and his special role of talking with authority to patient and family about the disease process, about prognosis and about grief, maintains his ultimate clinical responsibility and has no need to feel his *amour propre* insulted.

The chaplain or appropriate minister of religion may be needed for spiritual support with the authority of the church or faith he represents, to listen to confession and to give reassurance of forgiveness. It is not unusual for patients and families to find new understanding and help in sacrament and service. He also has a special importance as a listener, as has the social worker, just because they are people on whom the patient is not physically dependent.

The social worker tries to enable the patient and the family to understand and handle the problems with which they are faced. By listening and by her encouraging independence she can show patients that there are still decisions for them to make and a contribution to give in a situation where it is easy to feel they are constantly taking. The sorting out of the practical problems such as finance, community services and housing and the necessity of putting one's affairs in order can be turned into a means of marshalling the practical and emotional resources of the patient and of his family. By working with rather than for the patient, and by listening rather than talking, the social worker helps to maintain his self-respect as well as solve his social problems. Her work reminds the family and also the caring team that the patient is still a person who should be consulted and involved with family decisions whenever possible.

The physiotherapist has two goals: the maintenance or restoration of the patient's physical independence and the prevention of deformities which will curtail this independence. To keep a patient mobile or to get him to walk again is to raise his morale and self-respect enormously. To need to ask for everything, even if it is no further away than the locker, is to lose a basic independence which many patients find almost unbearable. It is irrelevant that this independence may not be long-lasting, and the physiotherapist as well as her patient must view achievement lost and gained on a day-to-day basis. The second part of the physiotherapist's work is to prevent deformities occurring; if deformities are allowed to occur, unnecessary stress and discomfort and unnecessary difficulties in carrying out nursing procedures will make the last weeks of a patient's life a time of increasingly painful dependence. Part of the skill in controlling physical distress in advanced malignant disease is to use drugs in such a way that the patient is still mentally alert and that, even if there is pain on movement, it is tolerable. If this is achieved the physiotherapist can often continue her work until the last day or two of life. There are other patients who find massage and passive movement or instructions about relaxation most helpful.

The occupational therapist, and sometimes the speech therapist, if they are people of enthusiasm and imagination (interested more in day-by-day progress than in long-term rehabilitation) will help to maintain the physical dimensions of a patient's life as long as possible (Weisman, 1977). The value of opportunities to be creative cannot be over-estimated and diversion may be the best pain reliever of all.

The basis of good terminal care is good nurses and its apex is a good ward sister. The latter must be a skilful and sensitive leader. The former must have come to some sort of terms with dying and with death, and have learnt not to hurry.

Remission

Admission can be turned into a welcome by courtesy and the emphasis on the patient as a person. The pains of dying and death can be alleviated by care and knowledge. Sometimes, however, between admission and death an unexpectedly long time may elapse. It is here that more than technique is required. This time can be hard for the patient, for the family and for the staff. It can be a time when each day has to be got through as best one can and when it may seem that death would be a merciful release. But in retrospect, this time of waiting often turns into a time of deepening relationships within the family and sometimes what can be called 'spiritual growth' in the patient. To have shortened such a patient's life, denying him and his family this time, would be a tragedy.

Patients who survive longer than expected become focal points in the ward to whom other patients and the ward staff can relate. They take their place with the orderlies, the volunteers and the families as essential parts of the working ward team.

Care of the dying calls for great flexibility on the part of the caring team. Although the emphasis has shifted from cure to care, the condition of the patient must be constantly reviewed and reassessed. If symptoms are properly controlled or the disease process slows down or enters a stage of remission, the patient may well experience a new lease of life. If the family have had their confidence restored and have had a rest from constant nursing, they, in turn, may be able to look after the patient again at home.

Patients who have been labelled 'terminal' must still be constantly assessed by all members of the caring team for potential improvement in their physical and mental well-being. Further active treatment may sometimes, and surprisingly, be indicated. Palliative radiotherapy, palliative cytotoxic therapy, antidepressant drugs or steroids may produce dramatic improvements in patients for whom no further active treatment had been considered appropriate. Such an improvement may well enable the patient to return home and enjoy valuable extra time with his family. The patient himself should be encouraged to treat the ward as if it were his second home from which he can go out for the day or the week-end. Sometimes his symptoms will be sufficiently controlled and his family sufficiently rested for him to be discharged home. Such a discharge will work only with the co-operation of the patient's general practitioner and his staff, the involvement of a domiciliary service (if there is one) and the assurance to the patient and to his family that should the home situation break down in any way readmission can be arranged immediately. For him there can be no waiting list.

This constant reassessment of the patient in the context of his family and the regular reviewing of the rate of progress of the disease itself calls for careful and regular clinical observations and consultation with all members of the ward team. It may also involve visits from or to a consultant in another discipline.

Management of dying and death

The moment of death is rarely unexpected and therefore the nurses will have had time to prepare the relatives. Young children are not usually present but teenagers should not be discouraged if they wish to be there. A nurse endeavours to join them at the time of death or to watch if for one reason or another the family cannot be there. It is she who draws the curtains and gently tells the relatives when death has occurred. This is a hard moment as death to them is often not obvious. The relatives around the bed almost always accept the offer of the simple set prayers which are then said by one of the nurses. For some families this offer is obviously unsuitable and it is not made without thought.

After death the relatives may well wish to be left alone behind the curtains. When the time is right the nurse takes them to a quiet room and gives them a hot drink and sympathy and sometimes just silence. Special customs or cultures will be respected.

The remaining patients in the bay are told of the death. As they will have witnessed the dying it will not be too much of a shock to them, but again they must be given time to react and express their own grief or fears.

When the relatives are ready to leave, the ward staff will have checked on the home situation, availability of friends and transport. At this moment a bereaved person should not have to return to an empty house.

A time on the following day will have been arranged for the family to collect the death certificate and property. This is an important occasion. Reception should inform the ward staff that the relatives have arrived and the ward staff should be responsible for greeting them and taking them to the visitors' quiet room. Refreshment should be offered and after some conversation the death certificate is handed over and clear instructions given on how to get to the Registrar's office and what will happen there. On this visit, funeral arrangements and any other immediate problems can be discussed. The doctor, the social worker, the chaplain and the funeral director should all be available if necessary. Should relatives wish to see the body this should be made as easy as possible and a nurse they already know should accompany them.

Many relatives wish to go back and see the remaining patients in the bay. Indeed they will sometimes continue to visit regularly, a fact which underlines some of the advantages of not hiding away the dying person. At St Christopher's Hospice, relatives will be invited to come back to the monthly 'Pilgrim Club' where they can meet with members of staff and sometimes with patients whom they have known during the time they have been visiting the Hospice. The ward staff will make it clear that if any problems arise the family can ring for help. 'Key person cards' (see Fig. 4.1) are completed for each patient, enabling the social worker to assess the relatives at risk as well as those who may just welcome a telephone call.

In-patient management in advanced malignant disease demands that the specialized knowledge of symptom control now available is used successfully. With symptoms controlled, the patient is freed, if he so wishes, to contemplate both living and dying; the family as a whole can come to terms with the truth; they can be grateful for all that has been good and say goodbye—not necessarily in words. Sadness will not be removed but bereavement may be lightened.

'Tranquil talk was better than any medicine;
Gradually the feelings came back to my numbed heart.'
Po Chu-I, 1946

References

ABRAMS, R. D. (1974). *Not Alone with Cancer*. Charles C. Thomas; Springfield, Illinois.

MELZACK, R. (1976). The Brompton Mixture: effects on pain in cancer patients. *Canadian Medical Association Journal* **115**, 125.

MOUNT, B. M. (1976). The problem of caring for the dying in a general hospital; the palliative care unit as a possible solution. *Canadian Medical Association Journal* **115**, 119.

PO CHU-I (1946). *9th Century Chinese Poems*. George Allen & Unwin; London.

SAUNDERS, C. M. (1973). The need for inpatient care for the patient with terminal cancer. *Middlesex Hospital Journal* **72**, 125.

SAUNDERS, C. M. (1975). Terminal care. In: *Medical Oncology*. Ed. by K. D. Bagshawe. Blackwells; Oxford.

WEISMAN, A. D. (1977). The psychiatrist and the inexorable. In: *New Meanings of Death*. Ed. by H. Feifel. McGraw-Hill; New York and Maidenhead.

A Comment: Nursing the Dying Patient

Peggy D. Nuttall

Dr West has described many practices which may be regarded as being part of the nurse's province. In so doing he has demonstrated the fact that, in the team devoted to caring for the dying, there may well be role reversals. Well established teams will be quite familiar with this situation, and few problems are encountered in this respect. However, for those nurses who are working in acute wards where the team approach is not the usual one and where the physician or surgeon is the prescriber of treatment, the care of the dying can present formidable problems.

In 1976 the Representative Body of the Royal College of Nursing unanimously passed this resolution:

'That this meeting of the RCN Representative Body, aware of the nursing profession's deep concern that many patients with intractable, incurable and terminal illnesses are experiencing considerable suffering which could be relieved by appropriate care and intelligent use of drugs, requests Council to approach all appropriate bodies (medical colleges and other associations) with a view to discussing methods by which better care provision can be made for these groups of patients.'

Three examples will serve to illustrate, in some measure, the feeling of frustration which exists among many nurses:

'I almost despair of improving the situation until doctors are given more training and experience in the speciality. Many seem unaware of the patients' distress and are unwilling to prescribe adequate analgesics until the last moment' (Nursing sister).

'As one who works in the field of terminal care in the community, one thing strikes me again and again. It is that, while nurses are interested and on the whole eager to learn and practice better terminal care, the medical profession is, in many instances, so far unaffected by development in this field. One suspects that this may be that the doctor is trained to cure at almost any cost, and regards a dying patient as a failure with whom he is unable to communicate' (District nursing sister).

'I believe that there has to be some re-education towards the terminally ill and indeed towards death among medical and nursing staff and the general public' (Community nurse).

The difference between the orientation of most doctors and the motivation of most nurses which reflects their different modes of education is not always appreciated. To many doctors death presents itself as a defeat. Nurses on the whole take a different view; their prime aim is usually care of people and the outcome of any illness is seen less in terms of pathology than on the effect that the illness is having on the patient's life. This attitude is strengthened by the fact that it is the nurses who have to maintain a 24-hour contact with the patient and his relatives while medical intervention is necessarily episodic.

The ward sister has no control over her own work-load; this will be determined by the medical policies of the doctors. If she has insufficient resources, in terms of time and staff, to provide the support that she believes patients and their relatives need, she will become frustrated. If additionally she thinks the patient is being deprived of effective therapeutic regimens which should be more generally available, her frustration may deepen into anger. The community nurse who is working with several general practitioners only some of whom may be interested in terminal care, will also be placed in a situation which can sometimes border on a real professional dilemma for her.

Situations like these provoked the Royal College of Nursing's resolution quoted earlier.

An important nursing maxim is to anticipate the patient's needs before he is aware of them. This can be achieved only by close, personal observation, attention to detail and intelligent anticipation of his reactions. It also requires a mature judgement to decide when encouragement is needed for the patient to perform a task for himself and when it is preferable to relieve him of the burden of making a decision.

The patient himself will have preconceived, and usually stereotyped, concepts of the roles of the various members of the therapeutic team. As he gradually sees the roles blurred he will more readily relax as he finds himself surrounded by people, all of whom have the same aim. It is well recognized among nurses that patients tend to relate more easily to members of the domestic staff, whom they see performing tasks they understand, than to the professional staff who carry out largely incomprehensible activities. Only when he sees for himself that everyone is prepared to 'bother' and to be bothered on his behalf, will he really relax.

No nurse will pretend that this is an easy atmosphere to achieve in a busy, acute ward. But a measure of success can be achieved if the whole ward team—from doctors to ward orderlies—can be aware of the situation. However, it does involve that most difficult of exercises, an alteration of attitude.

Dr Parkes, in discussing the question of 'distancing' (which features more prominently in the training of nurses and social workers than it does of doctors), writes: 'Human relationships are dangerous. When we get attached to our patients we begin to suffer with them . . .' (Chapter 4). This is something which must be appreciated, especially by senior nursing staff. There is a price to be paid by all who are continually in contact with the dying. Staff themselves need an outlet. This may take the form of a less involved listener—a social worker, a chaplain—or it may need a short break or change of duty.

'Distancing' is seldom possible for the district nurse. Not only is she in direct contact with the patient and unable to plead distraction by other patients, but she is also in close proximity to the family and others caring for the patient. Unlike her hospital colleagues, she is seldom able to appeal to a number of doctors, i.e. if the houseman fails to meet need, the registrar and consultant are there. For the district nurse, if the general practitioner is a weak support, her dilemma is often acute.

Nursing the dying needs the highest skills. The nurse must be deft, dextrous, observant, vigilant and sensitive to the needs of her patients and their relatives. She must be approachable and receptive to spoken and unspoken needs. She must recognize that she cannot respond equally to every patient while remaining aware that the 'unpopular patient' deserves as much professional skill and compassion as any other patient.

Nurses and doctors in a busy ward will often avoid the dying patient, passing his bed swiftly and reducing social contact with him and his relatives. The ward sister must be alert to such a situation and correct it. The nurses will take their cue from her but, if the medical staff continue to avoid the patient, the doctor–nurse relationship in the ward will deteriorate. The ward sister needs the support of her medical colleagues if she is to help her patients by making full use of the measures which now exist to relieve distress in the final stages of disease.

11

Out-patient and Domiciliary Management from a Hospice

Barbara J. McNulty

Editorial note

At the Department of Health and Social Security National Symposium on Care of the Dying in 1972, Holford quoted statistics to show that between 1965 and 1970 cancer deaths occurring at home decreased from 37·5 to 33·5 per cent of the total. Yet, he reported, 'the consensus among writers on the subject seems to be that terminal care should take place at home', and this appeared to be the opinion of those attending the Symposium. Reasons for this discrepancy became apparent during the meeting and are illustrated in this chapter.

Where an illness has a foreseeable end, many families wish to look after their relative at home as long as possible (Aitken-Swan, 1959; Wilkes, 1965). Yet too many of them are left with memories of unrelieved distress which serve to enhance the public fear of this disease, the reluctance to embark on home care and to militate against its early clinical presentation, diagnosis and treatment. The pain and other distress revealed by the district nurses who carried out a survey for the Marie Curie Memorial Foundation (1952) were reported years later by Rees (1972) and Parkes (1977).

Death is essentially a family event, and there is some evidence that there may be a significant difference in the morbidity and mortality among surviving spouses and relatives who cared for the patient themselves and those who did not. The risk of the nearest relative dying within a year of bereavement was found to be twice as great if the first death had occurred in hospital (Rees and Lutkins, 1967). But if patients are to have good care in their own homes the doctor must be satisfied, usually after hospital treatment and assessment, that it is appropriate, that the patient himself wishes it and that the family is willing and able, with support, to do so.

The reports quoted above revealed a serious gap in such practice and, following the initiatives of other voluntary bodies such as the Marie Curie Memorial Foundation in the UK and Cancer Care in New York, from 1969 onwards a domiciliary service was based in St Christopher's Hospice with the support of the DHSS as a research and development project. This involved extensive consultation with the community services and was pioneered by the writer of this chapter, working with one of the Hospice doctors, with experience in general practice, alongside the family doctors of this suburban area. It was soon found that such a consultation service would be used freely and that the small team of visiting nurses was welcomed as an extra community resource. Its case load rose quickly to 60 70 patients a month. Other ways of bringing extra experiences and skills into the home are being developed elsewhere and some of them are described in the following chapters. This is also a popular subject for symposia and training courses among family doctors and those who work with them. The concentrated experience of the specialized teams is drawn upon widely and may supplement but should certainly never supplant the work of the general practitioner.

Much of the literature in this field comes from family doctors: that by Worcester (1935) remains a classic recently reprinted (1977). He represents all those who have made home care for dying patients their special concern over the years. Courtenay's short contribution traces some of the problems and possibilities of a long-established family practice. Many family doctors care for their own patients in cottage and small local hospitals. Where this is possible it has been ideal for patient and family alike.

General traditions and the new knowledge being developed may, we hope, reverse the trend towards hospital dying and enable more families to fulfil their desire to care for their relatives to the end in their own homes.

References

AITKEN-SWAN, J. (1959). Nursing the late cancer patient at home. The family's impressions. *Practitioner* **183**, 64.

HOLFORD, J. M. (1972). *Terminal Care. Care of the Dying.* Proceedings of a National Symposium held on 29th November 1972. HMSO; London.

MARIE CURIE MEMORIAL FOUNDATION (1952). *Report on a national survey concerning patients nursed at home.* Marie Curie Memorial Foundation; London.

PARKES, C. M. (1977). Evaluation of family care in terminal illness. In: *The Family and Death.* Ed. by E. R. Prichard, J. Collard, B. A. Orcutt, A. H. Kutscher, I. Seeland and N. Lefkowicz. Columbia University Press; New York.

REES, W. D. (1972). The distress of dying. *British Medical Journal* **2**, 105.

REES, W. D. and LUTKINS, S. G. (1967). Mortality of bereavement. *British Medical Journal* **4**, 13.

WILKES, E. (1964). Cancer outside hospital. *Lancet* **i**, 1379.

WORCESTER, A. (1935). *The Care of the Aged, the Dying and the Dead.* Charles C. Thomas; Springfield, Illinois, 1961, Blackwells, Oxford. Reprinted 1977, *The Literature of Death and Dying,* Arno Press; New York.

This chapter is based on six years' work in the Home Care Service at St Christopher's Hospice, London, where I led a team consisting of three nurses, a health visitor and a social worker, working alongside the community services already available to the dying cancer patient and his family at home. We had available at all times the advice of one of the Hospice doctors with experience in general practice and could refer back to the original hospital through her. We could also call on the services of a physiotherapist and an occupational therapist. Perhaps most important of all, we had the special care beds of the Hospice behind us should the home situation unexpectedly deteriorate. It is the knowledge that these beds are available which gives us, our families and their own doctors the confidence to try to hold a difficult situation at home. The aim of this home care team is to support the dying patient and his family in their own home for as long as they wish and to the last, if possible. Response in the local community has been such that this team forms a bridge—a liaison between the hospital consultant and the family doctor, between the hospital and the home. It also ensures continuity of care for the patient who is able to go home from the Hospice with a guarantee that he will be readmitted when he needs it.

My observations are based on six years' work with 1500 patients with terminal disease and their families.

The problems encountered fall into the following categories: medical and nursing, social and financial, and emotional and psychological. So wide a range of problems cannot be dealt with by any one person, hence the need for a team—but a team closely integrated with constant two-way communication. Each member must be able to contribute his insight into the situation and to draw upon the expertise of his colleagues and of the family doctor and his team, who remain involved until admission becomes necessary.

Why home?

In the United Kingdom the number of deaths from cancer in hospital is twice that of deaths at home. Many believe, in their concern for the patient, that only in-patient care can offer adequate control of the multiplicity of distressing symptoms which may accompany terminal cancer. I would like to pose two questions: what is in the patient's best interests? what is appropriate to his needs? The doctor may feel that the patient will be better off in hospital but the patient may feel differently. Patients who still hope for a cure will wish to persevere with every possible treatment; those who have understood the true nature of their predicament may well want to be left in peace. Most patients will have been ill for a considerable time and will have undergone a variety of investigations and diverse forms of treatment. As the hope of cure recedes, it is not surprising that a patient should wish to go home and return to his familiar surroundings where he feels more himself, so that he may face his deteriorating condition in that security.

There are no absolute criteria to help us decide whether a dying patient can remain at home; each case is individual. For instance, a single person living alone may well be able to manage if his financial resources are adequate or if he has attentive friends and neighbours; one less well endowed cannot. Poor home conditions do not always preclude home care. The home may fall far short of the ideal, the care given may not come up to our standards, yet in spite of inconvenience and in spite of discomfort it may still be the best place for a particular person to die. The patient's need for home and the familiar surroundings outweigh anything which a hospital can offer. The decision turns on the material circumstances and on the quality of the human relationships within the home. When assessing the suitability of a home for terminal care, one must look closely at who will bear the brunt of giving the care, and how it will be given—with love or with resentment.

A dying patient's best interests will be served if emotional as well as physical needs can be recognized and he himself be given some choice of the right place for him. He may wish to die at home cared for by his family, or to remain there until the last few days and then return to hospital to spare his family. The answer to the question 'Why home?' is that it is often the patient's choice, that hospital beds are needed for those who require active treatment and, because of ward pressures, are frequently inappropriate to the needs of the dying. Families need the opportunity to express their love and caring before it is too late and so gain a sense of achievement which can soften the bitterness of grief. Patients derive comfort from familiar surroundings and routine patterns, whereas in hospital they are to some extent alienated from their true selves and isolated from life.

Family fears

The emotional and psychological problems encountered with the patient and his family can be overwhelming. Any worker in this field must be familiar with the anger, bitterness and resentment, the denial, grief and fear encountered in patients facing death. It is not enough to note these responses: one must know how to meet them and how to lead patients and family through the anger of 'Why should this happen to me?' to the calmer waters of 'I know I am going to die. I'm not afraid now.' For the family the dawning realization of their coming loss clouds all life with sadness. Added to this is the anxiety of wondering whether they will be able to cope and the weariness of giving constant care. These burdens can be lightened by sharing with a sympathetic listener who can also give practical help.

Preparing the family

Dr Parkes (Chapter 4) has referred to the importance of time to enable patient and family to come to terms with what is happening. If the patient has been at home for some weeks, the problems associated with his deterioration are likely to have been faced and overcome gradually; if he is suddenly discharged from hospital towards the end of his life there may well be anxiety amounting to panic within the family. As Mrs P. explained, she very much wanted to have her husband home, but when she was told that, as there was nothing more that the hospital could do for him, she might as well have him back tomorrow, she felt frightened. If the hospital did not know what to do, how would she? She was afraid of not giving the tablets properly. She knew that a nurse would come to do his dressing but she did not know how to cope with a burst abscess which soaked through dressings and bedclothes in the middle of the night. Her constant anxiety communicated itself to her husband and he began sleeping badly and worrying so much that within a few days he had to be readmitted, leaving them both with a sense of guilt and failure. This collapse of home care might have been averted by careful planning and forethought.

Including the children

Many fears stem from ignorance or prejudice. 'I know he wants to come home,' said Mrs W., 'but I couldn't have him, could I? What about the children? It would be terrible for them to see their father getting worse, and they might catch something.' These children were 7 and 9 years old, well able to realize their father's condition and much needing to be involved. Daily contact with him throughout the last weeks of his illness in their own home was less damaging to them than a conspiracy of silence and exclusion. Fear of 'catching something' is a common phenomenon and can isolate the sick person and make him feel an outcast. His removal to hospital will emphasize his alienation from the family and confirm their fears. Children are more capable of withstanding the stress brought on by their limited understanding of death than mystery and implied abandonment (Feifel, 1977).

Adequate drugs

When relatives express fear that they will not know how to cope with an emergency, they usually envisage uncontrollable pain. 'I can cope with the nursing and with anything else,' said Mr H., a devoted husband who cared for his wife for many weeks before her death, 'but I can't stand to see her suffer: I can't bear to watch her in pain. If she stays at home she will suffer more than if she goes into hospital. So I'll have to let her go.' The fears expressed by Mr H. were not without foundation for at that time his wife's symptoms were out of control. He was to find during the remaining weeks of her life that, as her various symptoms were treated and the levels of analgesic drugs were balanced to her needs, she was able to remain tranquil and almost pain-free until the end. Family fears that a patient nursed at home is likely to suffer more pain than if he were in hospital have been borne out by several investigators (see Editorial Note). However, there is much more that can be done for pain relief, and in most cases home care can be as good in this respect as hospital care (see Chapter 5).

Essentials for domiciliary care

Continuity and communication

In the bewildering mass of people to whom a patient is exposed during the course of an illness, there needs to be one whose responsibility it is to pass on vital information. For the patient and his family to feel secure, they must have confidence that their doctor knows what is the matter and will tell them what they need to know. They must also feel sure that the various professional people caring for them will keep one another informed of changes in treatment. Not until then will our care have continuity (Chapter 1).

The case of Mrs Betty F. (aged 34) illustrates many problems. She was visited at home at the joint request of the gynaecologist, who at laparotomy had found an inoperable carcinoma of ovary, and of her family doctor.

She lived in a dilapidated prefabricated bungalow with her mother of 78 and Sharon, aged 12, her daughter with spina bifida whose father had deserted at her birth. The financial assets of this household were her mother's old age pension, and her own unemployment and supplementary benefits.

Betty was devoted to her old mother and her handicapped daughter. She knew that she was dying and was desperate to remain with them. The main problem in enabling her to do so lay in the co-ordination of the many agencies involved.

The family doctor knew only about the young mother. Sharon was cared for by the paediatric consultant and the old lady had refused all medical attendance. The overall situation was known to the district nurses and the home helps who came daily. They had little power to alter anything. St Christopher's Hospice was asked to make suggestions for the control of Betty's pain, which, it soon became obvious, was closely related to her anguish for her family. She was admitted to the Hospice briefly many times for paracentesis and reassessment of pain control, and during these months a firm relationship built up with each member of the family.

Sharon was supervised by a social worker from the paediatric hospital who was in touch with Sharon's headmistress; neither knew of her mother's illness. The old lady was known to the health visitor in her area as one of the hundreds of inadequately housed elderly people for whom she was responsible. She was also known to the welfare authorities who paid her old age and supplementary pensions and to the housing authorities who received her frequent requests for urgent repairs to the crumbling fabric of the house. None of these knew about her daughter's illness or of her granddaughter's handicap.

The first step was to contact all the agencies involved and arrange a meeting in order to pool knowledge and sort out responsibilities. Throughout Betty's illness, St Christopher's Hospice remained the co-ordinating agent, at the same time working together with the doctor and the district nurses. Between us we drew in non-statutory help: a local convent made regular gifts of food packages; volunteers shopped and escorted Sharon to hospital; private charities made small grants and gifts; Boy Scouts redecorated the living room; a holiday (the first in her life) was arranged for Sharon. The old lady finally agreed to see Betty's gynaecologist and her complete procidentia was successfully dealt with.

When Betty died, the grandmother was inconsolable. Sharon resented her protectiveness, withdrew into herself and became insolent and unco-operative. Not surprisingly, she looked elsewhere for companionship and love. It fell to the St Christopher's visitor to listen to the grandmother's constant complaints about Sharon and to her own distress. Sharon's needs were even more urgent. She was growing up a precocious adolescent, physically handicapped and not very intelligent. Because we had known and loved her mother she accepted our further intervention almost with relief. She was now 16 and had acquired a boyfriend, and we were able to advise her about the problems of her friendship with him. We helped in the discussing of plans for her marriage, helped with finding living accommodation and suitable employment.

The role of a Home Care Team in terminal care is not likely to be brief, nor is it cut short by death. It continues with those who are left behind.

Trained staff

Lack of time and experience

Most doctors or nurses have little training in how to talk, or indeed listen, to the family of a dying patient. Without some experience it is difficult to know how to be with a dying man without self-consciousness, letting him direct the conversation. Staff have not been taught how to pick up the subtle, half-concealed questions which will give the vital clue as to how he can best be helped. This kind of support is needed in the home perhaps more than anywhere. The hard-pressed family doctor and the busy community nurse are often not trained to give this kind of support nor do they have the time to give it. There is a shortage of specially trained medical and nursing staff in the community; and their time is sometimes wasted in activities which could be undertaken by less highly trained or differently trained people.

Terminal care is costly in terms of time, people and emotions. The very ill cannot be hurried, are quick to sense impatience, and are easily made to feel a burden if those caring for them seem pressed for time. Yet adequate time is essential, for nursing care may be heavy or patient and family may need someone just to sit and listen.

Twenty-four hour care

Week-ends and nights may be a nightmare to many families caring for a dying person. We are still far from giving full 24 hour National Health Service coverage to patients at home, though many areas are making great progress towards this goal. Once the surgery has closed and the telephone number has been referred either to a central agency or to another doctor, the patient is cut off from the familiar source of help, comfort and reassurance upon which he has come to depend. It has frequently been left to voluntary initiatives to give that continuity of care so much needed throughout the night as well as the day.

Some doctors, when they know that a patient is dying, will give the family their home telephone number even though they are off duty. This goes only part-way towards solving the problem, for the doctor needs his off-duty time. Various solutions between the two extremes of the single-handed doctor and the impersonal relief service include group practices with partners who take turns at being on call (sometimes with specialist nurses available at any time) and special teams consisting of doctors and nurses who share or even take over the care of the dying.

Drugs in the home

In hospital it is relatively easy to assess the patient's changing condition and drug requirements; at home it is more difficult. Patients on the whole are uncomplaining. If their pain is bad or their nausea incessant, they will assume that it is probably unavoidable. Daily reassessment of a patient's condition and reappraisal of his drugs are essential. If the medical attendant cannot do this he must ask for a report from the visiting nurse or a responsible member of the family. It is not enough to have a supply of the current drugs in the house—some plan has to be made to deal with predictable emergencies. If acute dyspnoea or severe haemorrhage are likely, the family needs to know that the necessary drugs are in the house, that they are allowed to give them or, if not, whom they may call upon to do so. It is the unplanned-for crises that have undermined the confidence of so many people in home care.

Financial difficulties and loneliness

Every family suffers financially when nursing a sick member at home. There will be increased bills of all kinds—heat, light, food and laundry. Financial help of some kind will almost certainly be needed. To the young married couple who have taken their grandmother into their home the extra laundry or heating, invalid delicacies and extra comforts can assume impossible proportions, and they may be forced to send her into hospital. The working single woman caring for an elderly father may have to stay at home so often that she is in danger of losing her job. Old age pensioner couples not only find it hard to heat and feed themselves properly but, both being infirm, find it hard to care for one another. Yet this group, perhaps more than any other, needs to stay at home. The Misses P., both in their 80s and unwell, were determined not to be separated or sent away. Since they were unable to get out and were often both confined to bed, they were entirely dependent on their neighbours. That one would shortly die from widespread malignant disease was understood by both but not alluded to. Their doctor and health visitor deplored the situation but agreed to support it though they could not have managed if it had not been for the kindly neighbour upstairs who unobtrusively took control. Many people who are nursing a dying relative at home need increased financial help and befriending in a dependable and supportive way.

Some services available in the community

There are a number of agencies giving help of various kinds to patients in their own homes, but this help is all too often unco-ordinated and the agencies may be working blindly. Many people are unaware of the existence of such help and even their doctors are not always certain what is available.

Nurses

Most general practitioners now have nurses attached to their practice; these nurses may be privately employed or they may be seconded from the local authority. A few areas have a comprehensive 24-hour nursing coverage, and most have a 'twilight nursing service' or something similar, available through the nursing officer responsible. The Marie Curie Memorial Foundation makes funds available to local authorities for the purpose of employing night nurses to care for the terminally ill cancer patient, and there are, in some areas, Marie Curie trained nurses for night care.

Health visitors and social workers

More and more group practices have health visitors and/or social workers attached but, if not, they should be contacted through the local social services or in the hospitals.

Home helps

This service supplies women for general domestic help in the home. They give aid in many ways and much personal support. The local organizer should be contacted at the social services centre. Availability varies from area to area, and there is a charge to the recipient.

Nursing aids

Bedpans, urinals, ripple beds, hospital beds, bed cradles, commodes, etc., are available in limited supply through the community nursing services.

Laundry

Incontinent laundry service and the collection of offensive *contaminated dressings* are organized by the local social services, but the availability of such services varies from area to area.

Colostomy, ileostomy

Urine drainage bags and catheters, colostomy and ileostomy bags are prescribable on the National Health Service but have to be ordered and can take weeks to obtain. Patients discharged from hospital must be given an adequate supply.

Sterile dressings

These are available on National Health Service prescription but special requirements may take time to obtain and patients discharged from hospital should be given a good supply to take out.

Financial aid

The Attendance Allowance must be applied for on a form available from the Post Office and is available to families who are giving day and/or night time care to a patient at home. There is a six months' qualifying period and for this reason not many patients with terminal disease have been helped in this way.

The National Society for Cancer Relief makes financial grants to enable a patient to remain at home, and for extra comforts.

The Department of Health and Social Security have discretionary powers to give supplementary benefits and to make grants in exceptional cases. Application should be made to the local manager.

Social services have wide powers to supply funds for special needs such as adapting a house or putting in a chair lift. They may also be able to rehouse a patient.

Voluntary organizations

The Red Cross can sometimes help by sitting with a patient, with shopping or transport. Local branches should be contacted.

Cruse is a national organization for counselling and support to the bereaved. Contact should be made with Cruse House, 126 Sheen Road, Richmond, Surrey TW9 1CR, or to the local branch.

The Society of Compassionate Friends is a national organization for befriending and supporting parents who are facing the death of a child. Their address is 50 Woodway, Watford, Herts.

Other addresses

The Colostomy Welfare Group, 38 Eccleston Square, London SW1.
The Ileostomy Association, Drove Cottage, Fuzzy Grove, Kempshott, Basingstoke, Hants.

The Multiple Sclerosis Society, 4 Tachbrook Street, London SW1.
All three give help and support to families and patients with relevant problems.

The Disabled Living Foundation, 346 Kensington High Street, London
W14, can be of help with ideas and appliances for the chronically sick.

Local church groups can often supply companionship, befriending and
practical help both before and after a patient's death.

A helpful pamphlet, 'What To Do When Someone Dies', is published by the
Consumers' Association.

The Church Army and the Salvation Army will collect and dispose of
clothes following death, a service which is of great help to the bereaved family
as well as to those who are in need.

Chiropody, physiotherapy, hairdressing and barbering are occasionally
available in the home and are much needed adjuncts to the well-being of the
patient.

A variety of home care schemes

Some of the many centres specializing in the care of patients with advanced
malignant disease in the United Kingdom and elsewhere give home care. This
chapter has been based on the experience of St Christopher's Hospice. Some
examples of other centres, operating in different ways, are given below.

St Joseph's Hospice, Hackney, London

The Home Care Programme at St Joseph's was started by Dr Richard
Lamerton in 1974 with the help of one of the Irish Sisters of Charity who have
run the Hospice since 1906. Dr Lamerton has built up his team from the
community nurses working in the areas round the Hospice. One nurse from
each borough has been seconded to him. This Hospice has a doctor-centred
team, based in a unit where beds are available to him and consisting of nurses
employed by each district. Patients are referred by their general practitioners, and those who are well enough are seen in the weekly out-patient
clinic for regular assessment of their changing needs. They are also cared for in
their own homes by the nurses and, when necessary, are visited by Dr
Lamerton or his deputy. A twilight nursing service is given and one member of
the team is available at night by telephone. Some general practitioners practically hand over their patients to the Hospice home care team while others
work with the team and continue to visit, reporting any alterations in treatment which they may have made.

The Macmillan Unit, Christchurch

The Macmillan Unit for Cancer Care came into being in February 1975
through the efforts of Dr Ronald Fisher and the National Society for Cancer
Relief, the first of its kind to be maintained as part of the National Health
Service. The 25-bed unit and the Home Care Service started simultaneously in
the same building and work in close co-operation with one another. The
Home Care Service is still evolving and changing as it identifies the needs of
cancer patients in the area. Referrals to the unit and to the Home Care

Service are through the general practitioner who remains in charge while the patient is at home, though the unit doctor may visit. The three Home Care nurses visit patients regularly and work closely with the general practitioner and the community nurses. Their primary responsibility is to ensure the continuity of care of the patients discharged from the unit and to get to know those who may eventually need admission. They deliver drugs prescribed by the unit doctor and ensure that these are being taken correctly and effectively. The team emphasizes the need for time with the patient and his family and, like the St Christopher's team, they are concerned with every aspect of the physical and emotional needs of the patient and his family. This concern is extended into the bereavement period.

St Luke's Nursing Home, Sheffield

St Luke's is a 25-bed unit which opened in 1971, started by a general practitioner (now Professor Eric Wilkes) who is Medical Director, and is staffed by general practitioners. Home care is not part of St Luke's programme though prospective patients are sometimes seen at home before admission. An unusual feature about St Luke's is its flourishing day centre, open daily, to which patients are transported by volunteer car drivers. The day centre offers its patients medical consultation and supervision, some nursing attention if necessary, chiropody, beauty care, occupational therapy, physiotherapy and a variety of amusements and entertainments. Ten patients daily can be accommodated in the centre, 8 of whom will be suffering from malignant disease and 2 from other long-term illnesses. Some of the patients will have been discharged from St Luke's wards; others will one day require admission. In this way a continuity of care is assured to patients, and the staff are able to predict to some degree when admission will be needed. Liaison with community doctors and other staff is good and a liaison community nurse sees all day centre patients to assess their suitability for the unit. She also makes occasional supportive visits to the home when necessary.

Hospice Inc., New Haven, Connecticut, USA

The inspiration for the organization calling itself Hospice Inc. came from an American nurse, Mrs Florence Wald. Because of difficulties in finding suitable beds in existing hospitals, or a suitable site on which to build, or funds to do either of these, the project started with a home care programme. In 1973 Dr Sylvia Lack, from St Joseph's and St Christopher's Hospices, was appointed Medical Director and the following year she and a small group of nurses, a social worker and a few volunteers began to give full-time care to patients dying at home. Although they often have to travel considerable distances to see their patients, the team meets regularly. A small office takes telephone enquiries, relays messages and acts as a centre. No hospital beds are available to the team but in 1975/76 62 per cent of their patients were able to die in their own homes. If admission becomes necessary for their patients, the team usually loses sight of them though liaison and co-operation with other doctors is developing. Hospice Inc. has imaginative plans for an in-patient unit and will shortly start building so the nature of its work will undoubtedly change and expand. This was begun against all odds, with little money, and through the determination of a small group of people working with patients in their own homes. It obtained bridge funding from the National Cancer Institute (see Chapter 15).

The same pattern is being followed elsewhere in the United States; for example, Hospice of Marin near San Francisco. There are now (in 1977) some 50 groups in the planning stage in the United States and a few already at work.

Summary

Caring for a dying patient at home, however difficult it may be, is not only acceptable but frequently is the place of choice. The patient is in familiar surroundings and the family are left with a sense of having done their best. Both the patient and his family may have had the opportunity to work through old quarrels and misunderstandings and together come to a quiet acceptance. There are, however, certain basic essentials for home care:

1. adequate, trained staff who are familiar with the special needs of patients with terminal malignant disease;

2. good communication between hospital and community and between all members of the team;

3. sufficient time for patients and families to be able to voice their fears, anxieties and difficulties to the staff;

4. a full 24-hour coverage, both medical and nursing, on an internal rota system;

5. foresight and planning so that adequate drugs are available for emergencies, and frequent assessment of the changing needs;

6. a bank of nursing aids available for loan at a moment's notice;

7. a day centre and an out-patient clinic for those who are well enough, with volunteer car drivers to ensure quick and easy transport;

8. quick and easy access to beds should admission be needed suddenly, with the possibility of discharge always in mind and the certainty of a continuity of attitude and care;

9. a follow-up service to the bereaved with help and support in starting life again.

Reference

FEIFEL, H. (Ed.) (1977). Death in contemporary America. In: *New Meanings of Death*. McGraw-Hill; New York and Maidenhead.

A Comment
The General Practitioner and the Dying Patient

M. J. F. Courtenay

The inception of the National Health Service in 1948 split the previously integrated pattern of medical care, separating the hospital from community care, and, by implication, making the hospital the 'centre of gravity', in spite of the fact that general practitioners still looked after more than 90 per cent of illness.

The rapid advances in medical technology which were applied in the hospital context reinforced this division, and encouraged the public to think that all good medicine was practised within the hospital walls. A collusive pattern arose in which patients and their relatives came to feel that only hospital treatment could provide what was best in medical care, while the doctors came to feel that anything which could not be cured was not their responsibility. General practitioners now felt that they were excluded from the hospital facilities, but were still expected to receive patients discharged from hospital, frequently without warning or discussion and often in a condition for which the community resources were inadequate.

The revolution in the control of infective conditions produced by antibiotics altered the relative prevalence of other conditions such as cardiovascular disease and malignant disease. As terminal care for malignant disease assumed a greater importance in terms of total medical care, it challenged the altered functions of the hospital; though these patients were not curable (and therefore considered 'unsuitable'), the patients and their relatives felt that they would receive only proper care if they remained in hospital. General practitioners were faced with a feeling that they were expected to send their patients to the appropriate consultants and receive them back only if those specialists failed to cure and therefore discharged the patient. As general practitioners were trained in hospital they mostly shared the current medical opinion that proper medicine was hospital medicine, and felt doubly denigrated by being clerks in the first instance and nursemaids in the second. The concept of the caring personal doctor nearly perished.

The situation was not helped by the fact that the district nurses were not working closely with the general practitioners on a day-to-day basis, although ever willing to do everything to help patients. Ironically in the light of one comment (Chapter 10) by a nurse who felt that 'many [doctors] seem unaware of the patients' distress and are unwilling to prescribe adequate analgesia until the last moment', other district nurses felt that general practitioners were too ready to give large doses of potent analgesics. The scene was set for someone to review the alleviation of pain in advanced malignant disease, and this came eventually from outside the National Health Service.

Whatever the future of special units for the care of advanced malignant disease, it is certain that proper analgesic regimens might never have evolved without them. The pain relief protocol of St Christopher's Hospice (as developed from St Luke's Hospital and St Joseph's Hospice) is now available for 'education of the profession'. The literature available which lists the various drugs which may be useful has shown that the medication must be arranged so that symptoms including pain should be prevented rather than just treated when they occur (Chapters 5 and 6).

This does present difficulties in treating the patient at home, since someone other than the doctor must be relied upon to administer the medication in the correct way while the doctor monitors the dose and the procedure. In case of sudden emergencies, the limits of the delegated responsibility must be sharply drawn, and the methods of calling assistance set out in detail. The home nursing service is the key to this kind of management, though the responsible person may have to be the spouse or other close relative. Fortunately, nursing resources in the community are usually good and when the nurse has dealt with special problems, there are other ancillary services to call on, such as night attendants, who may allow the relatives to get adequate sleep or prevent an isolated patient remaining alone. Even so, the help of good neighbours is often essential to adequate care.

Apart from this pioneering educative role, special units will probably always be needed in the foreseeable future. The demand for acute beds in a hospital service starved of adequate resources and the inappropriateness of keeping certain patients at home will leave a gap which can be properly filled only by a special unit. For the general practitioner there must always be a back-up in case domiciliary care breaks down, because either the patient or the relatives reach breaking point. Increasing anxiety often renders a plan of symptom relief ineffective—what will work in a special unit or hospital does not always work when the patient is constantly worried that he is not in a 'safe place'.

The general practitioner has an important role to play in the management of terminal malignant disease, but only if he has absorbed the necessary information and developed the necessary skills. These are gradually becoming more available, largely through the GP trainee schemes which have been established over recent years.

The first fact for the GP to realize is that the number of patients in an average practice likely to need such care is very small, so that although it may involve extra time for each case, the total work-load is not greatly affected. The second fact is that, once the GP has divested himself of the feeling that the whole exercise is one of failure, this kind of care can be immensely rewarding. The perennial anxieties over what to tell the patient and how to handle the relatives' wishes or how to conduct the management wither away, provided the doctor can allow them to talk out their anxieties, and can assure them that the control of pain will be maintained one way or another, even though this may eventually mean admission to a hospital or a special unit.

The more professionals involved in the care of one patient, the greater the problems of day-to-day communications. While ideally one doctor should be in charge, and may arrange a special system whereby nurses and relatives can get in touch with him while otherwise off duty (and here doctor-initiated phone calls can be immensely useful), it is probably adequate if the care is shared with one partner, so that they can share the daily decisions about management. The extra work is more than repaid by what the patient can teach about the last voyage of discovery. To be with another person by turns frightened, angry, fighting and denying reality is a training process in itself. The doctor needs to identify with the patient, and then stand back professionally to seek the best way to meet his needs. Paradoxically, the certainty of losing the battle allows the GP the greatest possible freedom in being the patient's personal doctor. While exercising the highest skills in symptom control, he is involved with the twin dreads of separation from loved ones and the fear of death itself which are in some degree common to us all.

The rate of deterioration itself is an important factor in deciding how the patient is best to be served.

The question of mortality itself must inevitably be faced by every GP who enters this type of relationship. It is not necessarily a question of religious or philosophical belief; it is more the conscious realization of one's own feelings about dying. It is not so much answers that are required but the need to remember Donne's words that 'no man is an island entire of itself'.

12

Terminal Care in the National Health Service

Gillian Ford

'She saw that it was a whole world. . . .
Whatever she looked at, however far away it might be, once she had fixed her eyes steadily on it, became quite clear and close as if she were looking through a telescope.'
   Lewis, 1956

'Not only 1 per cent but one person is a relevant statistic if it happens to be you or someone you love.'

Definitions and perspectives

The purpose of this chapter is to appraise the management of the final stages of malignant disease in the context of the National Health Service (NHS). For most people during most of their lives, the NHS provides care and cure for illness 'events'—either in hospital or at home. There are exceptions: for example, private medical treatment outside National Health Service hospitals is used by some patients; and a number of charitably run homes supplement NHS or local authority accommodation for those who, because of age or disability, need a sheltered milieu. Sometimes new developments in medical care are pioneered by university departments or other research institutes and these may bear a considerable treatment load before the NHS is able to take up the service commitments. Generally, such developments are absorbed as their value is recognized but occasionally the 'non-NHS sector' makes a sustained contribution to care or treatment or both. Terminal care is an important example. Of the 40 or so special units for those with terminal malignant disease only 10 are within the NHS although most of the others receive some financial support from health authority sources. Apart from information about those separate units which are devoted exclusively to the care of the dying, there is little knowledge of the nature and quantity of particular services for this group of patients; indeed, terminal care itself is difficult to describe or define precisely. Diseases other than cancer may be responsible for distressing and disabling conditions prior to death, and by no means all patients dying from cancer require the prolonged pain relief and symptom control which is part of the specialized management of terminal disease.

Nevertheless, it is commonly held by both the public and the professions that death from cancer is a prolonged affair, often painful, often accompanied by progressive physical deterioration. Many staff experience considerable difficulty in tackling the problems of pain, fear and grief. The special units for terminal care, which do not need to give preference to curative medicine, have cultivated the approach to death and dying which does not deny the fact of death but sees that its attendant woes, whether of body, mind or spirit, receive attention and care.

Size of the problem

The gradual elimination of sudden and early death from infectious diseases has thrown into prominence deaths from neoplastic disease. These now amount to about 120,000 each year in England and Wales—or one-fifth of all deaths. The age/sex breakdown of deaths from all causes and from cancer is shown in Table 12.1, and the rates in Table 12.2. Death rates from cancer, as from all

Table 12.1   Deaths from all causes and from neoplastic disease, England and Wales, 1973

	All ages	0–4	5–14	15–24	25–44	45–64	65–74	75+
All deaths								
Male	296 546	7 802	1 494	3 346	9 791	75 899	95 605	102 609
Female	290 932	5 704	903	1 421	6 238	43 483	67 137	166 046
Deaths from neoplastic disease (ICD numbers 140–239)								
Male	65 406	172	297	345	1 981	21 689	24 765	16 157
	(22%)	(2%)	(20%)	(10%)	(20%)	(29%)	(26%)	(16%)
Female	55 891	124	196	242	2 422	18 037	16 391	18 479
	(19%)	(2%)	(22%)	(17%)	(39%)	(41%)	(24%)	(11%)

Table 12.2   Death rates per 100 000 population by age group and sex, England and Wales, 1973

	All ages	0–4	5–14	15–24	25–44	45–64	65–74	75+
All causes								
Male	1 240	77	37	96	158	1 337	5 151	13 635
Female	1 152	60	24	42	103	720	2 685	10 098
Malignant neoplasm								
Male	271	8·5	6·8	9·4	31	378	1 326	2 134
Female	219	6·1	4·5	6·6	39	295	649	1 114

Tables drawn from the Registrar General's Statistical Review of England and Wales for the year 1973 (HMSO, 1976)

causes, rise with age (apart from the 0–4s). The Tables show clearly that cancer deaths form a substantial proportion of early deaths (before 65), most marked in women aged 25–64.

The greater proportion of cancer deaths occur in hospital (Table 12.3). Deaths in NHS hospitals and at home account for close on 90 per cent of all cancer deaths—the remaining 10 per cent occurring in non-NHS hospitals or institutions or other accommodation such as private residential homes.

No strong trends are obvious from the figures for the last 6 years, but there is

Table 12.3   Total deaths and percentage of deaths occurring in non-psychiatric hospitals (NHS and other) and at home, England and Wales, 1965 and 1970–1974

Year	All deaths			Cancer		
	Total (1000s)	Non-psych. hospitals	Home	Total (1000s)	Non-psych. hospitals	Home
1965	549	50%	38%	107	60%	37%
1970	575	54%	33%	117	61·5%	33%
1971	567	55%	32%	118	63%	32%
1972	592	55·5%	32%	120	63%	31%
1973	587	55%	32%	121	63%	31%
1974	585	56%	31%	123	64%	31%

a tendency for more deaths to take place in hospital. It is not necessarily the case that as a result there is less care of patients in their own homes. Patients with malignant disease are spending less time in hospital for 'episodes' of treatment, and one possible explanation for this is that they are cared for longer at home even though death itself takes place in hospital.

The National Health Service

Historical background

At its start, the objectives of the NHS embodied the aims of the report published in 1942 of the Planning Commission set up in 1940 by the Royal Colleges, British Medical Association and Scottish Medical Corporations.
   These were:

   1. To provide a system of medical service directed towards the achievement of positive health, the prevention of disease and the relief of sickness.
   2. To render available to every individual all necessary medical services, both general and specialist, and both domiciliary and institutional.

The ensuing debate and protracted negotiations centred on the methods of provision rather than the aims, and the latter have remained essentially unchanged for more than three decades.
   The pattern of services provided in 1948 inevitably varied from place to place, not only because of the different level of capital investment in different parts of the country, but because perception of proper health functions was different between local authorities who were then responsible for providing community and personal health and social services, some of which now belong to the Area Health Authority. The 30 years or more which have passed since the original NHS Acts have seen far-reaching changes in the distribution of facilities and their administration. Following the recommendations of Seebohm,* Social Work Services were more sharply distinguished from health and became the responsibility of the local authority social services department as distinct from the local authority health department. The National Health

* Full title: 'Committee on Local Authority and Allied Personal Social Services'. Terms of reference: Appointed 'to review the organization and responsibilities of the local authority personal social services in England and Wales, and to reconsider what changes are desirable to serve an effective family service'.

Service Reorganization Act of 1973 brought together hospital and community health services under one area health authority, of which there are about 90 in England and Wales. Bringing the health services under one authority, by integrating the former tripartite administration, had the important objectives of reducing the gaps in care which could occur when one authority was responsible for one service (hospitals) and another when the patient was back in the community, and facilitating the planning of services for specific groups of patients who are extensive users of both hospital and community services, such as the elderly. The area health authorities and local authorities were brought closer together through sharing the same geographical boundaries, making joint action by health and social services easier. The policy of providing support services for the elderly in their own homes rather than admitting them to residential accommodation plainly needs the efforts of both authorities; providing services rather intensively for a period of weeks or perhaps months for the terminally ill patient at home may also need joint action by social and health personnel.

Regional health authorities (RHAs) plan and provide all the specialist hospital services, and every Region has at least one university hospital associated with a clinical medical school. These are foci for the development of the specialized work with a high content of technological expertise which used to be regarded as a London activity. Dependence on London for specialist services is much less marked now than in 1948 although 50 per cent of medical students receive their undergraduate clinical training there.

Hospital services for cancer

A number of different medical specialties may be involved in the treatment of patients with cancer at some stage during the course of the disease—general physicians and surgeons, radiotherapists, oncologists and clinical pharmacologists. The central core of specialist medical services is the district general hospital serving a population of the order of 100,000–250,000. Treatment for most types of cancer will begin within the district general hospital, with additional cancer services such as radiotherapy provided at a few centres in each Region. Concentration is economical of equipment and enables staff to sustain their skills, but one consequence is that patients may have to travel some distance if they are receiving regular radiotherapy as out-patients. This may be no more difficult than commuting to work, in the Thames regions, but the woman who lives in Hereford and needs radiotherapy may have to go to Birmingham for it. The annoyances of this have been partly eased in some places by building hostel-type accommodation so that patients can stay overnight without being admitted to a hospital bed. Treatment with cytotoxic drugs may be available in the same hospital as radiotherapy, but in only a few places are the cancer specialists grouped together in one department for the treatment of cancer and only two hospitals in England are entirely for cancer patients. There is, however, an increasing trend to co-ordinate the various specialties involved in cancer management. In some hospitals, teams of specialists from different disciplines come together to plan the individual patient's management throughout the course of his or her illness. This approach is particularly being developed in four NHS regions where experimental 'regional cancer organizations' (RCOs) have been established. The aim of these is to provide the highest standards of diagnosis and treatment for all cancer patients throughout the region. Medical staff in other regions will, no doubt, watch with interest the evaluation of the combined approach. The provision of terminal care facilities, their integration with general cancer services and the education of the profession in the particular problems of the patient with advanced cancer are important elements in the programmes of each of the RCOs. In Wessex Region, for example, a 25-bed unit has been built by the National Society for Cancer Relief in close association with the Regional Health Authority and the Regional Cancer Organization, and a consultant, who will be responsible for the continuity of care of the patient, has been appointed. He will be an essential member of each cancer management team. The more common pattern of cancer treatment, where the general surgeon first sees and treats the patient after referral and the radiotherapist is brought in later, reflects an 'episodic' method of tackling the disease. Well established methods of defining the patient's problems and of communication are necessary in order to establish an overall plan of treatment of both the neoplasm and associated symptomatic problems. Some centres have been set up in the United Kingdom for the treatment of particular types of neoplasm such as breast cancer (Guy's Hospital, London), choriocarcinoma (Charing Cross Hospital, London, and Jessop Hospital for Women, Sheffield) and leukaemias (Hammersmith and Great Ormond Street Hospitals, London). In the case of choriocarcinoma it was clear that the results achieved by staff with experience were very much better than those who had little or no experience. Such is the rarity of the disease that only a few units are needed. The disruption that treatment in distant units may bring to family life is bearable because of the strong chance of cure. General hospitals, including those which teach undergraduates, rarely have a section of the hospital set aside for patients who are terminally ill. This is generally deliberate policy to avoid part becoming known as a 'death ward'.* In some hospitals the medical staff decide that each member is responsible for the total care of his own patients from the time of initial treatment to the terminal stage, even if other disciplines are involved in clinical management during the intermediate stages. This often implies an undertaking to admit patients to the acute ward if symptoms or social conditions require it. Side wards or single rooms, where these exist, may be used for very ill or dying cancer patients, but clinical practice and personal choice vary; some patients do not like the additional physical isolation and the lack of distraction, while it places an additional burden, both practical and emotional, on the nurses. A small proportion of patients with cancer who are over 65 are treated in wards under the care of the geriatrician. Some general practitioners admit patients to small local hospitals near their homes. This may be necessary because constant nursing care or regular injections are needed, or because the family need a break from caring for the patient, or simply because neither patient nor family wants death to occur at home. General practitioners have the opportunity through postgraduate sessions to acquire the theory of terminal care, and some have studied the techniques at close range through courses organized in special units.

---

* The experience of the Palliative Care Unit in Montreal has not shown this to be so.

Community services

In some instances, patients will reach hospitals because the community services have carried out screening programmes such as those for cervical cytology or chest x-rays. More often, general practitioners dealing with patients whom they may regard as 'at risk' because of their age, way of life, or symptoms will have initiated the sequence which leads to hospital treatment and continuing surveillance. Both the community services run by the health authority and those of the local authority may be involved in the continuing care of patients in their own homes, with the object of sustaining the patient and his family. Home helps provided by the local authority may be assisted by volunteers from the Women's Voluntary Services (WRVS) (with 'meals on wheels') or perhaps the local church. The social worker may have a difficult and ambiguous role (Daniel, 1973) and, while not providing direct health care, may mobilize practical services, aids, money and offer general support to the family. The NHS primary health care team consists of medical and district nursing staff, and health visitors, and may be supplemented by Marie Curie Memorial Foundation nurses and other helpers, and by home visits from occupational therapists and physiotherapists.

Changing patterns of care

The face of the NHS has changed as a result of the gradual development of services in the provinces, and through administrative changes such as those which followed the (Seebohm) Report on the organization of social work services, and the National Health Service Reorganization Act of 1973. Equally profound development and technical advance have changed medicine itself in a number of important respects: not only have the scope and range of therapy increased, but there has been consequential growth of teamwork in providing care and increasing fragmentation of medical specialties as the sum of knowledge is spread amongst many individuals.

Even the words 'medical care' now require definition. Provided by doctors? Not necessarily. Including curative and supportive elements? Probably, although care is sometimes used as the term for treatment which is not directed at cure (see Chapter 1). It is some years since the general acceptance that 'care' provided by other health professions—nurses, physiotherapists, clinical psychologists—was complementary to that provided by doctors. The high standards of these professions, together with their own ethical codes and methods of enforcing them, place their members in the therapeutic team as a matter of right. Most teams have a leader and normally this will be its medical member, but increasingly the contribution to care of patients by the non-medical members has come to be recognized. Each member concentrates on what is naturally his sphere. Good nursing is not the presentation of a perfectly neat ward with patients in bed under immaculate counterpanes while the consultant and junior medical staff do their rounds. It is not the appearance of order, but the well-being of the individual patient which is accorded the highest priority. This may mean the patient is out of bed learning to drive a wheelchair or walking or anything else which retains independence (at a time not necessarily convenient for the grand round). It also means that pressure sores and constipation do not await the desultory attention which they might receive left to medical staff alone but are tackled by nursing staff bent on their prevention. The existence of the team is particularly important for the patient with terminal malignant disease in hospital. Even though active treatment may not be required, the skill of nursing staff and physiotherapist, the attention from the chaplain or minister and social worker will all combat the multiple ills and sorrows a cancer patient may experience. But perhaps the growth of teamwork is even more important for patients who are still at home. Although the proportion of deaths occurring in hospitals is about 60 per cent of all cancer deaths, a substantial proportion of patients die in their own homes while many more have spells at home before, or even during, the terminal stage. For them, the services which can be provided at home are invaluable. Nurses, home helps, 'meals on wheels', general practitioner visits may all be mobilized to provide care and support at home. Some other services are patchily available—a local authority laundry/incontinence service and night sitters.

The diversity of this community-based supporting team has its counterpart in the more purely medical skills concerned in treatment. Earlier, the different types of medical specialist concerned with cancer treatment and with terminal care were considered; any one of these may be the person responsible for the care of a particular patient at any one time—or possibly for the duration of his illness. The psychiatrist may also be involved. The separation of different specialties within the main bodies of medicine and surgery is not in itself a fault. It is an inevitable consequence of the development of medical knowledge, but it may have a marked effect on the service a patient receives.

Whether a patient is receiving care from a team which reflects the social and human factors recognized as important in treating ill health or from a team which is primarily medical but of different specialisms, certain weaknesses of team working have to be guarded against especially when the patient's diagnosis is cancer. A common problem for hospital staffs is that they do not know for certain who has been told what. Nursing and medical staff may be questioned and hope that their replies are appropriate for that particular question; the radiotherapist may be asked 'Did they take away all the ulcer?', the surgeon may be asked if plans can be made for a holiday. With the diffusion of skills and contacts between many members of the team providing treatment, it is possible that the patient feels that there is nobody in charge and this may become frightening if no more surgery is contemplated, a course of radiotherapy has just been completed and the patient is at home with sundry unpleasant symptoms. The general practitioner, if he has been kept in the picture about the various hospital treatments, now has an invaluable role. He can explain the rationale behind the treatment (or possibly explain it again) the side-effects of it, he can prescribe remedies for indigestion and multiple other symptoms with which the patient 'didn't like to bother the specialist'. Equally important, he can arrange for assistance from domiciliary health care workers, district nurses or health visitors and, as the situation dictates, from social services.

It may be the GP who realizes that the patient is suffering from more pain than he is prepared to admit during the course of a visit to out-patients ('it wasn't my usual doctor and they were all so busy. I know they've done their best and it seems ungrateful to complain that pain is still there even if it is in a different place'). Consultation on drug management between the GP and hospital staff or the possibility of treatment by a nerve block or referral to a hospital pain clinic may then result.

In many ways, treatment provided for *any* patient is tailor-made for that individual, whatever his diagnosis. But the straightforward conditions are so easily handled by staff and patients alike that a real effort has to be made to sit down and think what to do for the patient whose problems will only be partly alleviated, if at all, by further treatment directed at the cause, who is likely to need underpinning by social and health workers and whose family will need support and reassurance for an unpredictable length of time. Sadly, it is still possible that a patient's need for symptom or pain relief is not met ('they told me at the hospital that they couldn't give me anything stronger'). This is no fault of the NHS as a system of providing care, but the bigger the framework the more difficult it is for the individuals operating within it to remain in touch with each other and for a plan of management of the patient's problems to be developed and worked up by the different members of the team—hospital, domiciliary or both.

Home or hospital? Hospital or hospice?

The NHS combines community and specialist services in a unique way and there is quite a strong chance that patients with cancer may get the best that these can offer. Combining the elements of both takes patience and persever-ance, as a general practitioner well knows. Community care is not in itself necessarily better than hospital care. But because it is based on the patient's own surroundings, it is believed to be what he would prefer and so it will be unless he sees his family using all their energies, and more, in looking after him. Hospital specialist services are not necessarily less good at providing care than the community team, but the patient may not wish to be there (Chapter 11). Any precise policy laid down as to where terminal care should take place would be doomed to failure at the outset. It is not only a matter of clinical judgement; the patient's own circumstances and preferences will have a profound influence. Some staff feel that an acute general ward is not the ideal place to care for a dying patient because its pace and atmosphere are geared to the acutely ill person; the regular drug round may be held up by an emer-gency admission so that a four-hour interval is stretched to six, and few people feel prepared to discuss a patient's fears. Special arrangements such as an evening at home may seem trivial and burdensome to harassed staff—and patients are often reluctant to bring their own needs to staff busy with other patients. Nevertheless, the patient may welcome returning to a ward with familiar faces and routine, and indeed the majority of patients who die from cancer do so in ordinary wards in ordinary general hospitals, having spent varying amounts of time being actively treated in the same wards.

It is obviously important that, wherever a patient and his family decide is the right place for death to happen, there are staff who are experienced in dealing with the problems and symptoms of terminal malignant disease. This is not often taught in British medical schools as a subject in its own right. Nevertheless, it is being increasingly recognized that the surgical, radiotherapeutic or cytotoxic approaches are not the entire treatment, important though they be. The difficulty lies in appreciating that handling the human approach to the patient, after he has ceased to need the exercise of highly technical skills, is just as necessary as any other aspect of his treatment. This is not easy for anyone to teach and those who do it best may be the least aware of what they are doing. The specialist units provide students with a short but valuable introduction to the subject. Longer periods of study—the Joint Board of Clinical Nursing Studies course for nurses, residential or attachment schemes for doctors or students and other health workers—allow not only the principles of terminal care to be taught, but some chance of practising it. Perhaps the most important part of such teaching is that a student should recognize that it does not require a purpose-built environment, or a profound knowledge of pharmacology, nor is it an art to which many cannot attain. Given confidence and experience, it is possible that general practitioners would find they were able to keep more of their patients at home, but any trend to this would be matched by an extra load falling on the other domiciliary services—both health and social. The smaller families, more elderly population and working wives of today cannot manage death in the family without the help of others—be they trained personnel or neighbours. The medical and nursing professions recognize that the dying present problems which sometimes seem intractable. The future may perhaps see a build-up of expertise at local level; a unit, a team or perhaps a consultant with experience in the subject, whose skills could be drawn upon when the need arises.

Only comprehensive enquiries on attitudes and expectations will reveal the extent to which the NHS is meeting the needs of cancer patients and their families during the terminal phase of their illness. Studies such as those of Cartwright (1973), who looked at the lives and care of a random sample of adults who died, and Parkes' (1975) comparison of bereavement after deaths at home and in hospital and anecdotal evidence suggest that there are gaps which are most noticeable during the stages of illness when potentially curative therapy has ceased. The extent to which the special units have attracted local support suggests that they meet a perceived need and the question must be asked, 'Is it right that hospices continue to develop through charitable and voluntary sources, and does this indicate that the NHS is not coping?' This cannot be answered directly. The NHS has benefited much from the efforts of individuals who have concentrated on the needs of particular groups such as the blind. There is certainly an impression, despite many exceptions, that the NHS structure, the training and inclination of doctors and the other health care professions favour the systematic and technological aspects of patient care. This has left the development of some of those aspects of care relating to social, mental and spiritual well-being to people and agencies outside the NHS. But the essence of good care in terminal malignant disease, as in other spheres of medicine, is in the attitude of the staff who provide it, wherever they may chance to practise. The Royal Commission on the National Health Service (1976) concluded that 'The most precious resource the NHS possesses is the people who work in it and for it and the skill and application they bring to their work.'

References

CARTWRIGHT, Ann, HOCKEY, Lisbeth and ANDERSON, John L. (1973). *Life Before Death.* Routledge & Kegan Paul; London.

DANIEL, M. P. (1973). In: *Terminal Care. Care of the Dying.* Proceedings of a National Symposium held on 29 November 1972. HMSO; London.

LEWIS, C. S. (1956). *The Last Battle.* Bodley Head; London.

PARKES, C. M. (1975). Determinants of outcome following bereavement. *Omega* **6** (4), 303–23.

Royal Commission on the National Health Service (1976). *The Task of the Commission.* HMSO; London.

(Seebohm) Report (1968) Committee on Local Authority and Allied Personal Social Services. HMSO; London.

Addendum
Some New Developments

Cicely M. Saunders

A small, multidisciplinary 'Symptom Control Team' began to operate in St Luke's Hospital, New York, in April 1975. This group has no beds of its own and is called in by the physicians and their ward teams to see individual patients. They are also frequently consulted by the junior interns or housemen, with the encouragement of their seniors. The team members work alongside the ward staff and their help in thus solving ward problems together has led to their being accepted as a welcome resource. Lack of financial support has kept the team small and their case-load has remained at about 20 patients a month. One of the reasons for its speedy acceptance was the fact that several of their early patients benefited so much from the skilled control of their previous distress that, against all expectations, they were able to return home. A second reason was the ease with which the extra knowledge was incorporated into the ward practice. This method of working has great potential for teaching and practice, and the first such team in the United Kingdom is planned to begin operating on January 1st 1978 in St Thomas' Hospital in London. This is surely the most economical and direct way of tackling the problems of giving specialized care to a dying patient and his family in the wards of a general hospital and of sharing such experience in the most fruitful way.

Another approach was also developed in early 1975. A 12-bed Palliative Care Unit was opened in the Royal Victoria Hospital, Montreal, to care for patients with terminal disease in the Unit and in their own homes. The Unit had already completed a full programme of research (Editorial, 1976, Mount, 1976, Mount *et al.*, 1976, Melzack *et al.*, 1976) when in November, 1976, at a heavily over-subscribed conference on terminal care, Mount announced that the Unit had ceased to be an experiment financed by the provincial government and would henceforth be an integral part of the hospital (Shepherd, 1977).

The leaders of these two experimental groups have relied for training and information on several of the English Hospices, which in turn are learning from them.

In the United Kingdom, the National Society for Cancer Relief has frequently given support to the existing homes and hospices. This Society is now helping local groups to set up Continuing Care Units of 25 beds which are built on National Health Service (NHS) land and are maintained as part of the NHS. Most of these are developing in close liaison with the local doctors or with some form of domiciliary service. In some cases they are already being consulted by physicians in the local hospitals and are involved in undergraduate teaching. There is frequent interchange of staff and information between these units and those already in the field. There are other projects in the planning stage, developing alongside or within the NHS. Some are staffed by part-time family doctors but the Continuing Care Units and others are appointing full-time medical directors.

Their financial arrangements vary. Most of the older units and some of the new depend upon charitable sources for capital costs. Contractual arrangements with the Regional or Area Health Authorities cover the cost of maintaining many of their beds, at a lower cost than the NHS beds these patients would otherwise have occupied. While St Barnabas and St Luke's Nursing Homes and St Christopher's Hospice keep their costs to approximately 70 per cent of a teaching hospital and 80 per cent of a general hospital bed in their area, St Joseph's Hospice keeps the latter figure to 50 per cent. Each Hospice has a number of 'free' beds and a considerable financial gap to fill each year from gifts and donations. They normally have no private beds but some families wish to give something towards the care that it has given; for example, this amounts to less than 2·5 per cent of St Christopher's budget. Money has never brought a patient into the Hospice nor has the lack of it ever excluded a patient who needed its care. All these institutions owe a great debt to generous public support but spend little time in the usual methods of fund raising.

Separate units of this kind will demand considerable initial capital but there is no evidence to suggest that they are more expensive to maintain than the wards or units that are part of other hospital complexes. So far, they have found that their freedom has been encouraged by NHS interest and support and that this has made an important contribution to their morale and to the possibilities of pioneering new developments. Home care developments, in particular, have opened up a new dimension of terminal care. This care, in collaboration with the family doctor, may postpone admission or avoid it altogether (Chapter 11). The financial saving for the NHS would be seen to be even greater than appears from the comparative figures given above if the total cost of the treatment of many patients were to be calculated to include the time that they remained at home because their symptoms were well controlled and their families supported. But we are not only concerned with finances; the real value to a family must be expressed in human terms.

In spite of such voluntary enterprise and activity, most patients who die of cancer will die in general wards, and much of our endeavour should be directed to developments which can be made there. Wherever people die of cancer, they will need help at times from someone with specialized experience. Some of the essentials of good terminal management are more easily transferred than others. The control of pain and of other symptoms (Chapters 5 and 6) can be practised anywhere; indeed, some of the knowledge we still need concerning the specific causes of symptoms may be better elucidated in such a setting as a cancer hospital. Other components may be more difficult to work for and must be included in whatever way is suited to local circumstances and available staff.

References

Editorial (1976). Terminal Care: towards an ideal, *Canadian Medical Association Journal* **115**, 97–8.

MELZACK, R., OFIESH, J. G., MOUNT, Balfour M. (1976). The Brompton mixture: effects on pain in cancer patients. *Canadian Medical Association Journal* **115**, 125 29.

MOUNT, Balfour M. (1976). The problem of caring for the dying in a general hospital; the palliative care unit as a possible solution. *Canadian Medical Association Journal* **115**, 119–21.

MOUNT, Balfour M., AJEMIAN, I. and SCOTT, J. F. (1976). Use of the Brompton mixture in treating the chronic pain of malignant disease. *Canadian Medical Association Journal* **115**, 122–24.

SHEPHARD, David A. E. (1976). Terminal care: towards an ideal. *Canadian Medical Association Journal* **115**, 97.

SHEPHARD, David A. E. (1977). Principles and practice of palliative care. *Canadian Medical Association Journal* **116**, 522.

13

Discerning the Duties

G. R. Dunstan

Dying is a social activity, like being born. A report of someone being 'found dead' strikes a faint chill because—leaving aside occasions of foul play—it implies a being alone, unbefriended, neglected by the rest of us, in this last experience of life. Man is by nature social. As he is received, it is hoped, by welcoming hands at his coming into the world, so a hand—ministering, or friendly, or merely available—should attend his leaving of it. To discuss that attention in terms of duties detracts nothing from its humanity. 'Duty', like 'charity', has attracted the label 'cold'. The label is undeserved. To use the language of duty is but one means of knowing where we are, what we expect of one another, in a human relationship. Duty can be as warm as charity. It is useful to have it reasonably clear and understood as well.

Duty is mere debt: what we owe to one another. Some can give more, prompted by affection human or divine—affection, that is, for the person or for God in Christ overflowing onto the person. But duty can stand without affection. Sometimes it is better so. Doctors and nurses are men and women; if every clinical relationship were compounded with affection the strain would be more than most could bear. This is especially true in terminal care. Affection is proper to some human relationships; duty is proper to all. Duty is a formulation of apt responses to human claims.

The response is no less human for being dutiful. It is the more human as it is infused with the graces of an elevated, redeemed, humanity. Suppose that a patient is to be taken to hospital. In his sickness, in his helplessness perhaps and pain, he articulates a claim. The claim is met by an ambulance officer. His strict duty is to convey the patient to hospital with normal standards of care. If his personal response to the patient's claim is infused with courtesy, gentleness, a reassuring confidence and competence in knowing what to do and doing it, what to him is duty is to the patient more; it is a human relationship apt to his need, and he is comforted. They may never meet again. Yet something of eternal worth has passed between them, in terms of duty.

There are thus some elements in duty which can be prescribed; they can be stated as terms in a contract, explicit as between employer and employee, or implicit in an offer of professional service. These are duty's bare external features. Other elements cannot be prescribed; they can only be discerned. These lie at the heart of professional judgement. Where a discretion is allowed, where a choice is made or appropriate treatment decided, there the practitioner has to find or feel his way, within the terms of his general obligation.

He has general knowledge and experience to guide him—the accumulated wisdom of his profession, made his own by learning and by practice; he has a particular knowledge of his patient, his condition, circumstances, needs; he has colleagues to consult if he is in doubt; but his precise duty—what to do, advise or prescribe now—he can only discern, by a consideration of the empirical features in the light of his concept of the patient's interest or total good. As for the dispositions which grace the duty, those which the patient discerns and which, for the patient, lift the relationship above 'mere duty', these are hardly the practitioner's consciously to command; they become part of him as a result of a myriad choices and influences; they are his 'character', stamped upon him as by a seal upon cooling wax. They are beyond contract, beyond prescription; but they are real. Duty in its fullness is discerned.

The interests

The purpose of this chapter is to discuss the duties owed to the dying. First, however, we must expose the interests which the duties are to serve.

Dying matters to the patient. Rationally viewed, it will mean, when complete, an end to whatever suffering, pain, anxiety or undue dependency has troubled him in his illness. Considered, if at all, in terms of religion, dying may mean a passage to some new state, of waiting or expectancy it may be, or of purgatorial preparation or of enjoyment. What state is looked for depends upon the faith embraced. Few men with a religious conviction look upon death as the end. These are cerebral judgements, rational and religious. They possess some men in such a depth of their being as to create a great calm. Beneath are human feelings: in some, not far beneath; in many, dominating everything. At the level of feeling, dying means a severance with all that is familiar, relatives, friends, foes; a leaving of others with their mixture of griefs, regrets, freedoms, responsibilities.

Between life and death comes the process of dying. It holds many uncertainties. *Nihil certius morte, nihil incertius tempore mortis,** as men used to write when making their wills. Dying, viewed prospectively, is as uncertain in its manner as in its time. Rationally, men know that, given appropriate medical and nursing care, pain can be controlled. They know also that that quality of care is not yet available everywhere, and that death can still be painful. Judgement is further warped by talk of 'dying in agony', which used to attach to some illnesses inevitably, and which is still put about by the unthinking and by campaigners for euthanasia. It lingers in the mind. Men know, too, that if dying is protracted, there will be long dependency on others, whether at home or in hospital. Such knowledge, with its associations, brings emotion into play alongside reason. Reason and emotion may strive for the mastery; sometimes one may prevail, sometimes the other.

Instinctively man, as a biological organism, clings to life. Reason and emotion, locked in their own contention, may sometimes ally with instinct to preserve life; may sometimes, singly or together, go against instinct and prompt the ending of it.

Dying matters to the patient, therefore, principally because it puts him at

* Nothing is more certain than death; nothing less certain than the time of its coming.

the mercy of contending forces: between certainty and uncertainties; between human claims and obligations; between reason, emotion and instinct. The interest of the patient, therefore, is in the sort of terminal care which will enable him to reconcile and to override, so far as he may, that contention. This implies a wider care than one which concentrates only on the treatment of his medical condition or on the relief of its symptoms, important as both of these are. Duty begins with a recognition of the complex human interest, and with a gathering of resources to meet it.

Others beside the patient have interests. His immediate family and friends may be tied to him with the closest bonds of affection. They may need him, depend on him, emotionally, intellectually, physically, economically. His death may spell to them sheer loss. They may bear gladly the burden of his dependency, protracted though it may be: or they may grow weary under it, crave for relief, for freedom for other relationships and activities. His death, when it comes, may being this freedom, and perhaps, financial gain. Like the patient, therefore, they may be at the centre of a conflict. Their interest, then, is in such help and support as will enable them to come out of that conflict with integrity unimpaired and with human relationships undamaged or, if broken, reconciled.

Doctors and nurses have interests, involved with those of the patient and his kin. They have an interest in the advancement of their professional skills: their own personal fulfilment is involved in this in their awareness of work done as well as it can be done. They have an interest, not only in the integrity of their medical procedures and professional relationships, but also in an assured reputation for that integrity. When someone may benefit substantially from the patient's dying—or from his not dying at a particular time—his medical attendants must be free from all imputation of collusion. If public confidence in their integrity is weakened, the innocent will inevitably be suspected with the guilty, and vexatious litigation, and insurance against its cost, will grow.

Here are some of the interests to be served in terminal care. The related duties have to be discerned.

The duties

Of doctor and nurse

The terminal stage of an illness may be designated in terms of the patient's condition; it would describe the period when, with no prospect of remedy or remission, the only foreseeable course for the illness is towards the death of the patient. That designation would be matched in terms of the medical care offered; terminal care would be directed, not towards the cure of the fatal condition but towards the care of the person dying. This would be to serve his interest in achieving a good death when it is no longer possible to serve his interest in living a healthy life.

This distinction is crucial for the appropriate management of the patient. Surgical intervention may be called for in terminal care for symptomatic control, for the alleviation of distress caused by the progress of the disease. But if such intervention went beyond this necessity and purpose, it would not serve the patient's interest in dying; it would be an imposition which might have been justified in the preterminal stage, when remedial action was a possibility, but it would be inappropriate now. Similarly, the decision whether to administer an antibiotic drug to combat an infection would turn upon its purpose. If the purpose were to relieve a supervening distress, and if its action were specific to that end, then its administration could be appropriate. But if its purpose were to combat an infection (of the lungs, for instance) which, if left untreated, might result in an earlier and easier release for the patient than that to be expected from his primary malignant condition, then its administration could frustrate the patient's interest in his dying.

It is sometimes argued that there is no moral difference between withholding a remedy which would prolong life and taking active steps to terminate it—between 'allowing to die' and killing (whether from a compassionate motive or not is beside the point) (Glover, 1977). The argument does not carry conviction, certainly among practitioners actively caring for the dying, or among moral theologians (Mahoney, 1976). The critical questions concern the patient's interest and his corresponding right—that is, his claim upon professional duty. The interest of the terminal patient is in dying. The corresponding duty is to serve that interest, to assuage and support him in his dying. ('Allowing to die' is clearly an inadequate and pejorative misstatement of this course of action.) The withholding of the remedy is not therefore a negligent act (and to that extent culpable) but a deliberate one, chosen because it is matched to the patient's condition and interest (and to that extent without fault). The patient's right to die (which would be infringed by inappropriate intervention to prolong life) may not properly be translated into a right to be killed, nor into a duty upon someone to kill him. Any act directly intended to terminate life would be culpable, in respect of the patient because it would infringe his interests both in life and in dying, and in respect of the practitioner—be he doctor or nurse—because it would infringe his basic professional principle as a servant of life. It would infringe also the right of the public to be able to trust him and his profession wholly as such.

Confusion surrounds the middle course also, between management without intervention on the one hand and an action intended to kill the patient on the other. This course arises when it becomes necessary to administer analgesic drugs in such quantity that they may predispose to a pulmonary infection from which the patient might die. Advocates of euthanasia claim a moral equivalence of this action with the deliberate administration of a lethal dose; they do so in order to advance the proposition that 'doctors kill already', that the public expects them to, and that it were both more honest and more safe to give them a statutory licence to kill in defined conditions.

This argument is fallacious. It is in the patient's interest to have his pain relieved, and it is the doctor's duty to relieve it by appropriate means—those effective for the purpose, with the minimum of harmful side-effect. If the side-effect can be remedied by means consistent with the patient's general interest in dying, then there is a duty to use those means. In the case under discussion the analgesic drug is effective for its purpose. Control of pain may result in an improved general condition and spirits, and so prolong the patient's life. It may, however, predispose to a pneumonia which may shorten it. This would be a secondary effect, foreseeable as a possibility indeed, but not directly intended (though not avoidable) in the administration of the drug specific for the control of pain. Fault would not attend the giving of that drug, in law or in morals, no less drastic remedy being available. The intention is the control of pain, and this is the primary effect. A secondary effect, not intended, unavoidably accompanies the first. Moralists, on this account, are wont to cite the principle of 'double effect' in justification of the action; but the normal medical terms of 'appropriate management' are adequate to describe it (Duncan, Dunstan and Welbourn, 1977).

The withdrawal of intensive care may be considered in the same context. Switching off a respirator is not 'killing the patient', as it is sometimes said to be. 'Life support systems' are more properly 'function support systems'. They are used to support vital functions, either temporarily during surgical operations or temporarily after collapse in order to give time for spontaneous recovery of function, or for medical intervention to be organized, or to enable a clinical judgement to be made, whether spontaneous functioning will ever be resumed, or can be restarted, or not. To remove the support by switching off the apparatus is to give effect to a judgement that what is supported is not 'life' in the sense of an organic human activity controlled from the critical point of the central nervous system, the brain stem, but the functioning of organs, heart and lungs, already incapable of functioning by themselves because no longer in receipt of the appropriate stimuli from the brain. Their cessation, necessary (in the United Kingdom at least) for a clinical diagnosis of death to be made, is in truth the result of the cessation of internal stimuli, not of the withdrawal of external, artificial, support.

The propriety of such action can stand on the basis of normally accepted medical ethics. If ecclesiastical warrant for it is required, it may be found in an address of Pope Pius XII to a congress of anaesthetists in 1957, in which he stated when it is permitted, and when it is a positive duty, to withdraw the apparatus of intensive care. He placed such procedures in the category of 'extraordinary means' which, in contrast to 'ordinary means' of care, a patient is under no obligation to request nor a doctor to administer (Pius XII, 1957; CIO, 1965; Duncan, Dunstan and Welbourn, 1977). The argument, as before, can stand independently of the language in which it is expressed.

If, as has been said, the doctor's concern is with a person dying, and not only with a malignant disease, his duties will extend to the context of medical care as well as to the choice of care given. He may be faced with the question, whether to tell a patient of his prognosis, his imminent death, or not. Clearly, he should not lie, if only for the pragmatic reason that lying erodes our common interest in truth and so undermines trust; and trust is too precious, too essential, in professional relationships to be so put in jeopardy. May he, then, by whatever prudent and diplomatic means, withhold the truth?

To answer this question we return to the basis of our argument: the doctor's duty is to serve the patient's interest in his dying. Within that interest are possibly conflicting considerations. The patient has an interest, certainly, in being spared unnecessary pain, shock and anxiety; this could be served by a prudent withholding of the truth about his condition. But he may have other interests which require him to know; his affairs to set in order, his wordly goods to dispose of or assign, his debts to pay; some obligations to fulfil; some persons from whom to seek forgiveness, some perhaps to forgive, some with whom to seek reconciliation; and himself to prepare, it may be, for a new awareness of the presence of God. On grounds such as these he has an interest in knowing the truth of his condition (Edmund-Davies, 1973), of being helped into the truth (Mahoney, 1976). The conflicting interests in his nearest relatives may be similar. The doctor, therefore, has to discern his duty whether to communicate the truth or not to, and if so, how. Only personal and moral insight, gained from experience and matured in his own person, can help him to decide.

With the doctor in terminal care are the nurses and other ancillary staff. They stand nearer the patient than does the doctor; they attend him for a longer time, more closely and more intimately. They may therefore, from closer observation, contribute more knowledge of the patient (if not of the disease) than the doctor can attain. The doctor has a duty to respect that knowledge, to invite its communication, to be receptive to it; the knowledge ought to influence his decisions on apt or appropriate care. This same nearness to the patient can give rise to greater emotional attachment than the doctor has to experience; it should not be disregarded.

Of the patient's kin

If dying is the social event which we have envisaged it to be, the relatives and near of kin are involved with the patient in his dying. The main points of their involvement have been touched on already; so has the ambivalence of feeling to which that involvement can give rise.

There is a sense in which those relatives attending the patient put themselves under medical tutelage if not direction, in order that medical and family care can be concerted in the patient's interest. Yet there remains wide scope for initiative, for calm, imaginative energy, in the giving of appropriate support to the patient and his medical attendants. The quality of the interaction within the family group may affect profoundly the patient's well-being, and, therefore, the provision of medical care for him. The doctor may not subordinate his patient's interest to those of the relatives; but only a very shortsighted practitioner would act as though the relatives, with their own needs and feelings, were irrelevant to his patient's management. He has to take account of them for his patient's good. This mutual expectation, this reciprocity of duty, between the doctor on the one side and the patient-community on the other, needs more exploration than it is commonly given. Medical ethics are too often discussed in terms of the doctor's duties, what he may or may not do; that there are corresponding duties on the other side is generally forgotten.

Of the patient

The patient is in no condition to be lectured on ethics—his station and its duties. What he has not learned already, in the education of life, it is too late for him to learn formally in his dying. Yet there are other ways to discernment than instruction. In the long tradition of spiritual writing *De bono mortis*,* and of exhortation, *Disce mori!*,† there is assumed a duty to *make* a good death, to be

---

* On the good of Death
† Learn to die!

active in the management of it, not merely passive, a patient and nothing more.

The way to this is learned, discerned, in the interaction with him of the medical and nursing staff, his relatives and, if any, his priest. It would seem to lie in the right balance, if it can be found, of the active with the passive roles: knowing when to submit, certainly, and how to co-operate; but knowing also how to use the liberty given (when it is given) by relief from pain to attend to those inner recesses of being to which medical and nursing care may not penetrate.

An initiative is called for if personal obligations are to be met, affairs to be put in order, forgiveness to be sought and given, reconciliation to be effected. The initiative may cost effort, even pain. But the good relationship which is part of good terminal care may enable it. Death will come inevitably; a good death can only be achieved.

Of the priest

Every man is, in a sense, another man's priest, though the office is usually called that of the neighbour. It is to share the common human burden of mortality. It comes to one now: help him. It will come to you one day; you will welcome help.

There is also a special priesthood, derived from religion, from the common human faith in a relationship which transcends the human and is fulfilled in a divine being. This priest stands on the Godward side of man. He is a mediator of the things of God to man, and of the aspiration of man to God. He must act vicariously sometimes, saying and doing on behalf of men what he knows or must charitably suppose they would want to do and say for themselves. This office is called prayer, in its diverse forms. But, more than this, he is an enabler: he is to enable men to articulate themselves to God, to be themselves before God and so to offer themselves to God. This is his function, his profession, with the living, from childhood to old age. The supreme test of his art is in his ministry to the dying, his contribution to terminal care (Hopkins, 1880).

He is one of a community of care—those whom in this chapter we have seen seeking to discern their duties. He must find his place, and hold it, in this community, this team. He must learn to respect the physical, with all its demands, restraints and limitations: 'first that which is natural, afterward that which is spiritual', St Paul wrote, in a related context (1 Corinthians 15:46). Yet he betrays his office if he forgets his primary commitment to the spiritual, if he sees for himself no role other than those discharged by the social worker, or psychotherapist, or voluntary hospital visitor. His unique place is 'on the Godward side', his unique care τὰ πρὸς τον Θεόν* the things pertaining to God (Hebrews 5:1).

This care extends beyond the patient to the whole attending community. Always his must be an available priesthood (Dominian, 1970); always on offer; never withdrawn; never grudged or brooded over because not always accepted. This is expected of him, even by those who ignore or reject his ministry. And as he is accessible to others, so he must have access to a counsellor of his own. He cannot care properly for the souls of others without care for his own; that care he is under duty to seek.

* ta pros ton Theon

This is the office of priesthood. It has been written out of some understanding of Christian priesthood, just as the duties discerned, and the relationships, the forgivenesses and the reconciliations to be sought, derive from the Christian view of man and his calling. No apology is made for this; a man can write only of what he knows. If what has been written matches the need of men of other faiths, or of none, that is well. What is given is only what has been freely received. Were there no match, that would be sad. But the quest is open. Others may discern duties of their own.

Felix Randal

Felix Randal the farrier, O he is dead then? my duty all ended,
Who have watched his mould of man, big-boned and hardy-handsome
Pining, pining, till time when reason rambled in it and some
Fatal four disorders, fleshed there, all contended?

Sickness broke him. Impatient he cursed at first, but mended
Being anointed and all; though a heavenlier heart began some
Months earlier, since I had our sweet reprieve and ransom
Tendered to him. Ah well, God rest him all road ever he offended!

This seeing the sick endears them to us, us too it endears.
My tongue had taught thee comfort, touch had quenched thy tears,
Thy tears that touched my heart, child, Felix, poor Felix Randal;

How far from then forethought of, all thy more boisterous years,
When thou at the random grim forge, powerful amidst peers,
Didst fettle for the great grey drayhorse his bright and battering sandal!

Poems of Gerard Manley Hopkins

Third Edition, Geoffrey Cumberlege, Oxford University Press, London, New York, Toronto 1948.

References

CIO (1965). *Decisions about Life and Death*. Church Information Office; London.
DOMINIAN, J. (1970). An Available Priesthood. In: *The Sacred Ministry*, Ed. by G. R. Dunstan. SPCK; London.
DUNCAN, A. S., DUNSTAN, G. R. and WELBOURN, R. B. (1977). *A Dictionary of Medical Ethics*. Darton, Longman & Todd; London.
EDMUND DAVIES, Lord Justice E. (1973). *Proceedings of the Royal Society of Medicine* **66**, 533.
GLOVER, J. (1977). *Causing Death and Saving Lives*. Pelican Books; London.
HOPKINS, G. M. (1880). *Felix Randal*, see also *Times Literary Supplement*, 19 March 1971, 331.
MAHONEY, J. (1976). *The Way* (April) **16**, No. 2, 124–35.
PIUS XII, Pope (1957). *Acta Apostolicae Sedis*, 1027. French translation in (1966) *Ethics in Medical Progress*. Ed. by G. E. W. Wolstenholme and M. O'Connor. J. & A. Churchill; London.

14

The Law Relating to the Treatment of the Terminally Ill

Ian McC. Kennedy

That a book on the management of terminal disease should include a chapter written by a lawyer may seem odd. Surely, the argument goes, treating the terminally ill is a medical matter, properly and uniquely within the expertise of the doctor. The answer is that the law has something to say in this area just as in most other areas of activity. Doctors may resent what they see as the intrusion of law. Many have a stereotype of law as a body of irritating rules, insensitive and often irrelevant to their daily practice. This view is, however, ill-advised. In all areas of medical care, and the treatment of the terminally ill is a particularly obvious example, decisions are made and conduct engaged in which are based not on scientific but on normative principles. The very word 'management' in a medical context connotes a choice among alternatives—for example, whether to discontinue the administration of pain-killing drugs at the request of a determined but possibly confused patient. Such a decision is fundamentally a philosophical and moral one for which the doctor, though he may have had greater exposure to it, has no greater training or expertise than the layman. Being so, the decision should be made in the light of principles deemed appropriate by society as a whole. Thus the doctor must observe not only the rules of his science and his profession but also those of society. Laws are one form of society's rules. They differ from, for example, morals or ethics in that they have the distinctive quality of being thought sufficiently important to be backed by sanctions for non-observance. They set standards for the regulation of conduct which purport to reflect a general popular consensus.

It is one thing to say that in the abstract the doctor must operate within the law; it is another to particularize that law. One of the greatest difficulties which confronts the medicolegal commentator in dealing with the treatment of the terminally ill is that techniques and technology have developed and changed with such rapidity in the past decade or so that it is only vaguely that the *problems* are perceived, let alone responded to, by developing a general consensus in the form of law. Some general legal rules do exist, but they assume a set of medical realities long overtaken by events. The sudden realization by the courts that respirators and cardiac pacemakers had made a legal definition of death based upon the absence of vital functions outmoded is a good example. Further, whatever legal rules do exist largely with the conventional medicolegal issues of acute and emergency treatment and with malpractice. These rules are by and large irrelevant in dealing with the terminally ill patient who is, in a sense, in a special class. Such a patient is by definition going to die sooner rather than later, and the regimen of care adopted, overshadowed as it is by the mass of available technology, calls for distinct and very sensitive regulation. This regulation must take account of and seek to resolve one particularly intractable problem which bedevils all medicolegal discussions and is highlighted in the care of the terminally ill: the tension between the paternalism of the doctor and society and the right to self-determination of the patient. Traditionally, the law has been too ready to adopt as right whatever the doctor decides. Since the doctor's view can hardly be called objective and since the decision is philosophical rather than scientific in nature, legal rules must be developed which strike the appropriate balance between the two according to the general popular consensus. Of course, doctors resent this attitude. It smacks of distrust. They would say they are good doctors who always act in the patient's best interests. But society and the patient need to provide for the eventuality that the doctor is not a good doctor (and these do exist) and what is in the best interests is not always necessarily best answered by the doctor. Moreover, not only have legal rules failed to develop, but the concepts which provide the stuff of legal rules are equally ill-equipped to respond adequately. For example, a legal system which sees the contact of a doctor with his patient as an assault or battery made lawful by consent, and rests so much on the notion of informed consent without showing any real understanding of the dynamics of the patient–doctor relationship, is in danger of losing respect.

In the light of the foregoing I treat with some trepidation the invitation to spell out what exactly are the legal rules governing the treatment of the terminally ill. However, I will endeavour to do so in a series of propositions with explanatory additions where appropriate (Kennedy, 1976, 1977).

1. A patient who is conscious and refuses further treatment must have his wish respected, whatever his condition, provided he is mature and lucid enough to make such a decision. If the doctor thinks the patient is not sufficiently lucid or mature, then the decision should be ignored.

This stems from the proposition that any treatment which is administered without consent is unlawful. To abide by the refusal may be difficult for the doctor but is required by law, the principle of self-determination overruling any notion that 'the doctor knows best'. In the unlikely event that a patient in a hospital refused even nursing care, for example bathing or changing sheets, different considerations would apply. The hospital's duty to maintain hygiene and protect the health of other patients would entitle the hospital to demand acceptance of such care as a condition for remaining in the hospital. Continued refusal would justify discharging those patients fit enough to be moved and with somewhere to go, and forcing the others to submit. This does not extend to feeding a patient against his will which I regard as a form of treatment. Clearly, the basis of this proposition is whether the patient is lucid, that is, understands the nature and implications of the decision and is competent to make it. The final arbiter of this is, of course, the doctor. The decision is made harder by the knowledge that almost all terminally ill patients are receiving medication and suffering pain and distress, all of which could affect their mental competence, quite apart from the doctor's reluctance to withdraw treatment. Ultimately the good faith of the doctor must guide his actions since complaints after the event by patients or relatives may founder for lack of proof. Putting the patient's request in writing may guarantee that his wishes are respected and protect doctors from later complaint.

2. When a patient is near death, a doctor is not obliged to embark upon or continue heroic treatment which has no prospect of benefiting the patient.

An alternative, more common, term than 'heroic' is 'extraordinary'. It was Pope Pius XII (1957) who first advanced the view that doctors were not obliged to give, nor patients to accept, 'extraordinary medical measures'. The term has consistently been interpreted as meaning 'whatever here and now is very costly or very unusual or very painful or very difficult or very dangerous, or if the good effects that can be expected from its use are not proportionate to the difficulty and inconvenience that are entailed' (Church Assembly Board, 1965). An example of an extraordinary measure in the case of the terminally ill would be a respirator where the patient can no longer breathe for himself. In his 1976 Stevens lecture, the Archbishop of Canterbury (1977) expressed his support for this as a moral principle. I take the view that it is also the legal principle. Indeed, I would go so far as to say that a doctor who continued treatment past this point would be behaving at least unethically if not unlawfully.

3. A doctor's obligation, when he can no longer hold back the approach of death, is to make the patient comfortable, including easing his pain. If, to ease pain, the doctor must take measures which may hasten death, this is permissible, provided the doctor's aim is only the relief of pain.

This reflects the so-called double effect theory and was incorporated into English law in one of the few decided cases in this area, R v. Bodkin Adams (1957).

4. The relatives of patients have no right to make decisions on the patient's behalf unless the patient is incompetent. Even then, the relatives may only act in the best interests of the patient.

The incompetent patients are the unconscious, the mentally unfit and immature minors. The test for what is in the best interests refers to general societal values rather than the views of the particular relatives. Thus, for example, the refusal by a relative on the patient's behalf of further treatment need not necessarily be respected. To allow otherwise may enable unscrupulous relatives, purporting to represent the patient, to precipitate his death. Equally, a relative may not demand treatment be continued or altered if, in the view of the doctor, it is pointless.

5. The doctor may not embark on any conduct with the primary intention of causing the patient's death.

This would be homicide. Put another way, euthanasia (whether or not at the request of the patient) is unlawful. The distinction between killing the patient and terminating treatment to allow death to take place is sometimes a fine one and taxes philosophers and lawyers. Some see the distinction in terms of a commission which is unlawful and an omission which may not be. I do not adopt this distinction. Though it is part of the general law, I regard it as unhelpful here. The real argument is not how a doctor's conduct can be categorized but whether in the circumstances he has fulfilled his duty to the patient in good faith. The principles of good faith reflect professional ethics and general social morality. Neither at present condones enthanasia. Thus to cause the patient's death whether by omission or commission would be a breach of good faith and hence unlawful.

6. If a terminally ill patient expresses a desire to commit suicide, a doctor may not in law facilitate the suicide (Suicide Act, 1961). To do so would be a criminal offence.

For the majority of these propositions there is no authority in the sense of legislation or court decision. Though I am confident of their validity, it clearly is unsatisfactory for the law to remain a matter of conjecture. It follows that there is a need for some authoritative synthesis of the law. The form this should take is, in my view, a Code of Practice worked out by representatives of the medical profession together with lawyers, theologians, philosophers and other interested laymen. It would not be a statute but would serve as the authoritative guideline while retaining flexibility and being easier to amend. Two recent examples of the use of Codes of Practice are the Report of the Medical Royal Colleges and their faculties in the United Kingdom (1976) on the Diagnosis of Brain Death and the discussion document of the Royal College of Nursing (1976) concerning a Code of Professional Conduct. Breach of the rules laid down in the Code would give rise to charges of unethical conduct and could serve as strong evidence of civil and/or criminal liability.

References

CANTERBURY, ARCHBISHOP (1977). *Journal of Medical Ethics* **3**, 57.

Church Assembly Board for Social Responsibility (1965). *Decisions about Life and Death*, p. 52. CABSR.

KENNEDY, I. McC. (1976). The legal effects of requests by the terminally ill and aged not to receive further treatment. *Criminal Law Review*, p. 217.

KENNEDY, I. McC. (1977). *The Listener*, July 14, p. 42.

PIUS XII, Pope (1957). *Acta Apostolicae Sedia*, **49**, pp. 1027–33.

R v. BODKIN ADAMS (1957). *Criminal Law Review*.

Report (1976) Conference of Medical Royal Colleges and their Faculties in the United Kingdom: Diagnosis of brain death. *British Medical Journal* **2**, 1187–8.

Royal College of Nursing (1976). Discussion document: Code of Professional Conduct. RCN; London.

Suicide Act 1961, section 2.

15

The Philosophy of Terminal Care

Cicely M. Saunders

'The practice of medicine is an art, not a trade; a calling, not a business; a
calling in which your heart will be exercised equally with your head.'
    Osler, 1903

The Shorter Oxford Dictionary includes as definitions of philosophy—that
department of knowledge or of study which deals with ultimate reality, and
also, the study of the general principles of some particular knowledge, experience or activity. Both definitions have been used to cover the substance of this
book in the belief that, as in any field of care, we will only respond fully to the
second if we give heed to the first. Here we are concerned with the nature of
man, with living and dying, and with the whole man—body, mind and
spirit—part of some family unit, with physical, practical needs for us to tackle
with maximum competence.

The early chapters cover the development and natural history of malignant
disease and the underlying causes of the clinical problems which face the
doctor treating the patient whose tumour is no longer controllable (Chapters 2
and 3). Crucial decisions concerning appropriate treatment presuppose a
discussion of all information available, while changes in therapy call for
detailed adjustment to each individual's particular needs and circumstances
(Chapter 1). Skill in understanding and controlling symptoms make such
decisions easier to make. The alternative to 'all available treatment of the
tumour' is no longer seen as negativism or neglect, but as a demanding and
effective clinical discipline in its own right. The finely balanced therapies
considered in Chapters 7 and 8 may, at times, still be appropriate for patients
with far advanced disease but should more often be accompanied by the
supportive therapy discussed in Chapters 5 and 6. But the time comes for
many patients when the active measures have little to offer and it is to be
regretted that many patients die still enduring exacting 'active treatment'. Do
we wish to spend our last days in this way?

When the decision is made that this is no longer the right way to treat his
patient, the clinician turns to the control of any distress but there should never
come a time when he says that he has nothing more to offer. Recent advances
in elucidating pain mechanisms have not yet eliminated the need for the well
tried drugs for the last days of a patient's illness. However, we may look
forward to better understanding in this field, to more subtle employment of the

psychotropic drugs, new adjuvants of other kinds and to the possibilities of other forms of pain control. Sounder knowledge of the underlying pathology of hitherto intractable symptoms may also make their treatment more rational and effective. But even now, while 'intractable' may mean 'not easily dealt with' (Concise Oxford Dictionary), it does not mean 'impossible'. The approaches and regimens described in chapters 5 and 6 can bring relief now—with an assurance of success for the great majority and, with dogged persistence, substantial relief to the 'hard core' of 10 per cent or less reported in several studies (Melzack, Ofiesh and Mount, 1976; Parkes, 1977; Saunders, 1959, 1976).

The increasing knowledge of the underlying disease processes and the tested methods of relief which can and should always be given, form a large part of this book. Such knowledge has to be balanced with a detailed consideration of social and personal factors. 'Feelings are facts in this house' as one of the nuns of St Joseph's Hospice put it, and intuitive thinking has to be added to the discursive if we are to approach the full reality of another person. Much of what is written here is concerned with feelings, with emotional and family suffering. These have frequently been described as making up the complex 'total pain' (Fig. 15.1) which our patients have often endured before they come to us, though criticism has been made that this use of words carries the

'Total Pain'

Physical

Mental

Social

Spiritual

Fig. 15.1. Total pain.

suggestion that such negative emotions should be avoided at all cost (Proudfoot, 1976). The automatic prescribing of antidepressant drugs or tranquillizers is to be deprecated; grief is appropriate and the understanding of suffering and its creative handling may be as important as attempts at its alleviation. The use of the word 'pain' was a deliberate attempt to stimulate students and others to look at the various facets of a dying patient's distress, beyond the requirement for analgesics to the need for human understanding and practical social help. This does not preclude the use of such drugs, but it does put them into perspective.

As Carter and Calman give the pathological and clinical background for the major therapeutic sections of the book, so Parkes' chapter introduces the psychological and social problems discussed by West and McNulty. To balance their presentations of a specialized team approach, Ford, Courtenay and Nuttall underline the challenge of interpreting this within the practicable and generally available. This is not meant to imply that this knowledge can be derived only from St Christopher's Hospice; there are many other centres, old and new, to which reference has been made.

Some chapters may seem surprising for a medical textbook, but dying patients ask more than medical competence of their doctors. It is not only Mr A. 'Who happens to have terminal cancer' with whom we are concerned, it is also Dr B. 'Who happens to be looking after him'.

The use of words is always interesting. On more than one occasion, having given the title 'Dying, *they* live', I have found the poster says, 'Dying, *we* live'. And many years ago, I remember a patient reading the *Nursing Mirror* and finding my name under some such title as 'The Care of Terminal Patients'. She said, 'Doctor, I object! I'm not going to terminate, I'm going to die!' In one of those unpremeditated answers that are occasionally given to us, I found myself saying, 'But, Mrs T., it's your illness that is going to terminate, not you'. Since then I have not knowingly talked of 'terminal patients', only of 'patients with terminal illnesses'. Some believe that the end of the physical body with its burden of illness is the end of the person. Whether or not we believe this, we owe our patient our skill and our honour to the end.

'Wherever patients happen to be dying'

The preceding chapters have been written from individual and team experience and from widely differing backgrounds. Their suggestions can be put into effect wherever patients happen to be dying of cancer. Terminal care does not have to be carried out only in a geographically separate unit, though there are some patients and families who need the expertise and the space they should find there. A few hospices will be needed for patients with intractable problems and for research and teaching in terminal care, but most patients will continue to die in general hospitals, cancer or geriatric centres or in their own homes; the staff they will find there should be learning how to meet their needs.

The following list of the essential components of terminal care is the fruit of years of working in different units and of endless discussions with others working and interested in this field (Kastenbaum, 1976; Wald, 1976). Above all, it is the outcome of the good fortune which gave me the opportunity of listening to patients and their families during the 30 years since that first patient told me that he wanted 'What is in your mind and in your heart'.

Essential elements in the management of terminal malignant disease
Concern for the patient and family as the unit of care

Families should have every available option open to their choice and expect recognition of their cultural and individual needs. Once this has become part of the ethos of a ward it appears to be largely self-perpetuating but occasional visits by ward staff to a patient's home with a family doctor or a domiciliary team member will emphasize the importance of including the family in the care of any seriously ill person. Not everyone will have the time or the understanding to embark on long family discussions, but everyone can recognize the family by name and accept them as an integral part of the team caring for the patient (Chapters 4 and 10). We should aim to give the maximum of privacy to those who need it for peace and for the expressions of tenderness which are inhibited in a general ward. Separate units usually have more opportunity to give a special welcome to the solitary but I have often seen how nurses in a general ward are able to do this and to make the distinction between the lonely, who welcome their friendship, and the isolated, to whom this may well be an intrusion. Here too, children can be welcomed.

Management by an experienced clinical team

The team or unit for terminal care must carry out its practice in such a way as to earn the respect and co-operation of the doctors who refer their patients. A multidisciplinary medical approach is as important in the later stages of cancer management as in the earlier phases of the disease. Consultation will often be needed between physician, surgeon, radiotherapist, chemotherapist and sometimes the psychiatrist and the clinician who runs the local Pain Clinic. It is no longer adequate medicine to try to cope alone with difficult decisions in terminal cancer management, even though the needs of many patients have been and still will be dealt with successfully by their own family doctors single-handed.

A group of consultants in a unit or team may act merely as a resource while the patient remains in the care of his family doctor or of the specialist who was involved with his initial treatment. The team may, however, take over his treatment completely, particularly if there is some special need such as intractable physical distress, intense family involvement in looking after the patient or the welcoming of young children to be with their dying parent easily and informally. There need be no feeling of rejection if transfer to a special ward or hospice is carefully discussed and planned; but whenever the original doctor keeps in touch, his visits are likely to have a special place in maintaining a patient's morale. Few patients expect miracles at this stage but they are all prone to feelings of failure and rejection, and respond to a gesture that implies continued concern.

Expert control of the common symptoms of terminal cancer, especially pain in all its aspects

Doctors and nurses need to concentrate on the development of these skills and special units should initiate research and combine their knowledge. Terminal pain is so different in character and meaning to most pain met in a teaching hospital that the methods of giving relief and the standards of comfort and alertness which should be expected are sometimes difficult to establish in a general ward. This has to be demonstrated to both doctors and nurses if their patients are to have adequate treatment for the many symptoms that often accompany this usually generalized disease (Chapter 6). They must also be helped to become aware of the mental and social aspects of suffering (Chapter 4).

Skilled and experienced nursing

Qualified nurses having short periods of training will gain and also contribute in a team of more permanent staff (trained and untrained) who maintain stability and continuity in the ward. This demands confident leadership from the ward sister and close communication between the nursing staff and all the others who will be involved with their patients: social workers, physiotherapists, occupational therapists and of course the doctors (Chapter 12). A flexible staffing pattern cannot easily be established in a general ward and lack of time is a constant problem. This can be exaggerated; an attitude can be conveyed in a brief meeting or in the way in which procedures are carried out. Student nurses frequently bring their special contribution in such ways. The chaplain's place in the whole team may begin from his support of the nursing staff who, most of all, bear the daily burden of relationships with dying and sorrowful people.

An interprofessional team

This is not the field for total individual involvement, which can be most unhelpful for both patient and staff member. It takes time to build the way of working described in Chapter 10 but such teams are to be found in other specialized units—for example, Intensive Care and Renal Dialysis. They are particularly needed by those who are grappling with emotional as well as with practical demands. Psychiatrists and social workers have frequently been involved as support. Volunteers may have an important role in the team.

Such a team, together with all its professional members, should be seen to include the ward orderlies, domestics and porters, often the people to whom hospital patients turn to most easily. Their support should not be underestimated or ignored. Students of all kinds may also assume this role, being themselves low on the pecking order, for the patient frequently feels that he himself is at the bottom. It is important that as many different members as possible meet for frequent discussion. Though the clinician does not abrogate his clinical responsibility, each member should be ready to assume a degree of leadership concerning an individual patient or family.

A home care programme

A home care programme must be developed according to local circumstances and be integrated with the family practices of the area and the in-patient unit. Patients can then be admitted at the moment of their choice and of accurately defined medical need, and they will also be able to move easily to and from the wards for periods varying from days to weeks or months as short-term improvements are fully exploited. Confidence may enable a family to keep a patient at home, often confounding all predictions. Where patients have access to adequate nursing, a 24-hour call service and other support, which may well include good neighbours, home is likely to remain their choice. Even so, many people who have said they would like to die in their own homes need in-patient care, if only for the last few days. Some families find much greater relief and unity in a professional milieu in the last hours and others realize that they cannot face the thought of death at home after all.

Bereavement follow-up

Many hospitals make special arrangements for families who come to collect certificates and property, but our work should not end there. The family has to recover. A bereavement follow-up will identify and support those in special need, working in co-operation with the family doctor and any local services which can be involved. Many doctors give such support as part of their service to the families they have known over the years. Some of the bereaved are not so fortunate and a follow-up as described in Chapter 10 may fill this gap and ease the tragedy and long morbidity of some bereavements. Social workers and chaplains have initiated such work from general hospitals, but normally a team as described in Chapter 11 will be required to meet with all those in need, with a leader to train and support the visitors themselves. There is no doubt that many families suffer from the sudden break from the people who have cared for the patient and have perhaps for a long time been a great part of their lives. In a small unit the families will be recognized as they enter the door and reception staff have a special role in this part of care for the bereaved. An informal welcome back may be all that is needed. It has been found that only a small proportion of the bereaved will remain dependent upon this support for more than a few months.

Methodical recording and analysis

Recording such as is described on p. 12 makes possible the evaluation and monitoring of clinical experience and the establishment of soundly based practice. Research in basic science, pharmacology and therapeutics and in psychosocial studies is needed to define and refine our practice and our attitudes.

Hinton's important study (1963) of the physical and mental distress suffered by 102 patients in the general wards of a teaching hospital is a definitive work and an essential reference point. He has since made other valuable contributions (1964, 1974). From the enormous volume of writing now available, we can still turn for enlightenment to the pioneer work of Worcester (1935), who published the lectures he had been giving to the medical students of Harvard from his background of family practice. This classic is still in print (1977) but gradually the anecdotal approach is being supplemented by the more analytical. Review articles such as Saunders' (1967) would now be almost impossible such has been the volume of writing since then. Conferences of those who are active in the work further the exchange of views on practical problems at local, national and international levels, and give encouragement to those who feel that they are battling against much inertia and opposition. This is a challenge to those who feel that 'tender, loving care' is all that is needed. Nothing can take its place, but terminal care of the 1970s developed from and should not now be the same as that of the 1900s or even the 1950s. 'Efficient loving care' is our aim and—as this book shows—every resource of clinical and social medicine has to be exploited.

Teaching in all aspects of terminal care

Teaching in this field is much in demand by students and graduates of all the disciplines concerned. This is given in conferences and seminars, in lectures and ward rounds and as in-service experience, both within the units and in outside visits by members of the staff. We find that any lectures and ward rounds of this kind are likely to be overcrowded. However (in spite of encouraging comeback, often years later, from those who have attended only one session), there should be reinforcement of such teaching for medical and nursing students in their own hospital wards. One of many groups of medical students who visited St Christopher's Hospice at their own request wrote afterwards: 'It was a relief to be able to discuss freely a subject which is usually actively avoided in a large teaching hospital'. Though much of the future development must be more closely integrated with general teaching centres, the special units are likely to maintain their role of stimulating initial interest and organizing courses for those who will in their turn be concentrating in this field. This is no longer a discipline in which no past special experience need be required.

Imaginative use of the architecture available

There should be space for families, windows for patients to look from, and opportunities for them to move around; room for staff to work easily and to relax; and 'transition spaces' for the anxious to take time off or to brace themselves for a meeting. Above all, a feeling of openness to the world outside and good public transport are chief among the needs of a unit for terminal and long-term care. Some of us have been fortunate enough to plan purpose-built units, others have learned to adapt whatever they could find, and successful practice has often arisen from the imaginative use of structural peculiarities. Emphasis should be given to the need for spaces for private talk; these must be found, whatever the area offered.

The proportion of single rooms to bays or wards dictates the way a ward team handles the patient's last hours and the needs of his family at that time. Some feel strongly that no patient should be expected to witness the death of another person dying in the same room or bay. Others, mainly those with fairly generous space and windows, find that this can usually be managed so that the reaction of most patients and their families is almost entirely positive. The peaceful death of a patient who shows no distress in breathing or in any other way, who is not left alone and, above all, one who is not hidden behind screens and curtains, repeatedly enables other patients to feel more confident about their own end. A distressing death would indeed have the opposite effect but those who are expert in such care should not let this occur. Families in the bays talk with each other and with other patients and it is rare for them to return for the practical business of the next day without going to see those they have known (Chapter 10) to give thanks for the friendship that has comforted them both.

Longer-stay patients play a special role in the life of a ward as part of its hospitality and support although, like the staff, they will need a holiday from it at times. Patients admitted within a very short time of death and certain others will require single rooms. As St Christopher's Hospice enlarges from 6 single rooms in 54 beds to 18 single rooms in a total of 62 beds, it has these groups specially in mind. It also looks forward to the day when it can enlarge its residential and half-way house accommodation.

A mixed group of patients

Although the homes or hospices which welcome only dying patients have given superb care for many years and by doing so, have frequently outweighed any fear locally of a 'death house' yet we do not believe that this should now be the ideal. A good community is usually a mixed one.

In 1958 St Joseph's Hospice had 150 beds, of which one-third were kept for patients terminally ill with malignant disease. The other patients were either long-stay, of various age groups, or the frail and elderly. Throughout a long rebuilding programme it has reduced its beds to 120 and has started two new developments of hospice care. Its Domiciliary Programme (Chapter 11), developed 'for anyone who happens to be dying in the area', is closely integrated with the hospital and community services of a part of London which often has slender general practice cover. It has recently opened a resource centre for those with long-term handicapping disorders, and offers short-term residential treatment and resettlement facilities. These programmes are revolutionizing the attitude of families in the area to the Hospice.

St Luke's Day Centre (Chapter 11) and most of the new Continuing Care Units include a proportion of patients with non-malignant diseases of a longer-term nature. St Christopher's Hospice has welcomed 10–20 per cent of its patients from this group, and a group of elderly people who live in their own bed-sitting rooms. Transfers to and from the wards are fairly common and there is no doubt that the Hospice will extend its longer-term accommodation of this kind when it becomes possible. The person with the prognosis of some two years often has more difficult problems to handle than the one with only some two months to live.

The Marie Curie Memorial Foundation Homes have welcomed patients for convalescence or for hostel accommodation while undergoing radiotherapy. St Luke's Hospital, Bayswater, London, has recently changed its name to Hereford Lodge and now offers longer-term convalescence, holiday and emergency admission to those being nursed at home as well as care for patients with advanced cancer, who now occupy only half the available beds. Hospice care is not limited to those who are dying but may be offered to all those who need more personal and less technological care than is usually easy to give in an acute general ward. It takes place in all the special centres mentioned, while Cottage and Community Hospitals have long concerned themselves with such work (see Chapter 11).

An approachable central administration

Efficiency is very comforting, and competence in administrative detail gives security to patients, families and staff. It also eases the liaison with outside contacts that is so essential for the small, specialized unit.

Members of staff will become drained by the work of the wards and in other contacts with the families of patients, and some are at risk of developing what has been described as the 'staff burn-out syndrome' (Freudenberger, 1975). Informal safety valves should arise spontaneously according to local personalities and surroundings but care must be taken to see that not only regular off duty but study leaves and extra time off are arranged before a crisis is reached. Staff members must be prevented from investing all their emotional commitment in their work.

The search for meaning

The work will at times cause pain and bewilderment to all members of the staff. If they do not have the opportunity of sharing their strain and questions they are likely to leave this field or find a method of hiding behind a professional mask. Those who commit themselves to remaining near the suffering of dependence and parting find they are impelled to develop a basic philosophy, part individual and part corporate. This grows out of the work undertaken together as the members find that they each have to search, often painfully, for some meaning in the most adverse circumstances and gain enough freedom from their own anxieties to listen to another's questions of distress.

Most of the early homes and hospices were Christian foundations, their members believing that if they continued faithfully with the work to which they felt called, help would reach their patients from God. Some of the traditional ways of expressing this faith are being interpreted afresh today and there are also many people entering this field who have still to consider their own religious or philosophical commitment. This is not an optional extra; it has a fundamental bearing on the way the work is done.

In considering these essential components of terminal care it is important to distinguish between the general principles being interpreted at St Christopher's Hospice and its own peculiar characteristics, stemming from the personalities of its staff and, above all, from its Christian foundation. The seed from which the Hospice grew was a gift of £500 left by a man from the Warsaw ghetto who died of cancer in a London hospital in 1948. His promise, 'I'll be a window in your Home', was fulfilled 19 years later when the first patients were admitted. That phrase and his other request, 'I want what is in your mind and in your heart', sum up the need of all patients for the skill combined with friendship that make up terminal care. The original gift of £500 had grown to £500 000 when the Hospice was opened in 1967. Now, 11 years later, the need to extend further its research into the control of pain in all its aspects and the ever-increasing demands for teaching have grown far beyond its original ideas; but they must still be balanced to the daily needs of each patient, family and staff member.

Many are convinced that the time and manner of this beginning and growth were the work of the God who said, 'My grace is sufficient for thee: for my strength is made perfect in weakness' (2 Corinthians, 12:9). Our confidence in this grace has grown as we have seen that the patients have always been the central members of the community. Every day they bring their pain and their feelings of anger, bitterness and grief into the Hospice as they are admitted. Yet the overwhelming majority find the atmosphere is peaceful, welcoming and often joyful, and their pain and many of these feelings are transformed. We believe this is the work of the spirit of the God in all men, however they may seek for truth and interpret the meaning of their lives in response to 'the true Light, which lighteth every man that cometh into the world' (St John's Gospel, 1:9) St Christopher's Hospice, whose founding patient and present Chairman both belong to the Jewish faith, is yet fully committed to the belief that, in Jesus of Nazareth, God knew a human life and the ultimate weakness of death as we know them, and this for all men, whether or not they yet believe. 'In all their affliction he was afflicted, and the angel of his presence saved them' (Isaiah, 63:9). Only a God whose love fully shares all pain from within can still our doubts and questions, not because we can understand but because we can trust. There is a sense in which we say, 'This is His Body' of each dying person and in which the small transformations that we witness continually speak of a Resurrection which will finally redeem and encompass all creation. This is the edge of that unsearchable abyss of deity which we meet in our daily experience, the beyond in our midst.

It seems to us that only the belief that all men belong to the family of a God who shared and shares their death can bring an answer, not only to those whom we try to help but also to the millions of the deprived and wronged; not only to those who face their end with peace and fulfilment but also those who have never had any chance of finding either a worthwhile life *or* death. That all wrongs will be righted and all the comfortless comforted should be the perspective of the individual, personal care that is offered in a hospice.

This is also the perspective in which the St Christopher's Hospice staff say to those of different beliefs or of none, together with the atheist doctor and the priest in Camus' novel, *The Plague*, 'we're working side by side for something that unites us—beyond blasphemy and prayers' (Camus, 1948).

References

CAMUS, A. (1948). *The Plague*, Hamish Hamilton; London.

FREUDENBERGER, H. J. (1975). *The Staff Burn-Out Syndrome.* Drug Abuse Council Inc.; Washington DC.

HINTON, J. (1963). Mental and physical distress in the dying. *Quarterly Journal of Medicine* **1**.

HINTON, J. (1964). Editorial. Problems in the care of the dying. *J. Chronic Diseases* **17**, 201.

HINTON, J. (1974). The influence of previous personality on reactions to having terminal cancer. *Omega* **6**, 95.

KASTENBAUM, R. (1976). Towards standards of care for the terminally ill. Part III. A few guiding principles. *Omega* **7**, 191.

MELZACK, R., OFIESH, J. G. and MOUNT, B. M. (1976). The Brompton Mixture: effects on pain in cancer patients. *Canadian Medical Association Journal* **115**, 125.

OSLER, W. (1903) *The Master Word in Medicine.*

PARKES, C. M. (1977). Evaluation of family care in terminal illness. In: *The Family and Death.* Ed. by E. R. Pritchard, J. Collard, B. A. Orcutt, A. H. Kutscher, I. Seeland and N. Lefkowicz. Columbia University Press; New York (awaiting publication).

PROUDFOOT, W. (1976). Commenting on 'Living with dying', Saunders, C. M., *Man and Medicine* **1**, 246.

SAUNDERS, C. M. (1959). *Care of the Dying.* Nursing Times Reprint. Macmillan; London.

SAUNDERS, C. M. (1967). *The Management of Terminal Illness.* Hospital Medicine Publications; London.

SAUNDERS, C. M. (1976). *Care of the Dying*, 2nd edn. Nursing Times Reprint. Macmillan; London.

WALD, F. (1978). Report of International Work Groups in Death, Dying and Bereavement: proposed standards for terminal care. In press.

WORCESTER, A. (1935). *The Care of the Aged, the Dying and the Dead.* Thomas; Springfield, Illinois. 1961, Blackwells; Oxford. Reprinted 1977, *The Literature of Death and Dying.* Arno Press; New York.

Index

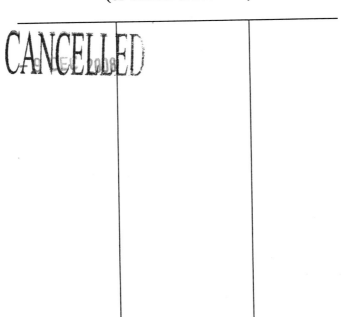